WALL PILATES *Workouts* FOR WOMEN

– WEIGHT LOSS EDITION –

Melt Away Pounds and Embrace Your Best Self by Slimming Your Waist and Pushing up Your Booty with Step-by-Step Illustrated Full-Body Exercises

AURORA POWERS

TABLE OF CONTENTS

STRETCHING EXERCISES

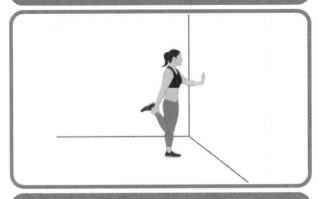

Page 11

CORE EXERCISES

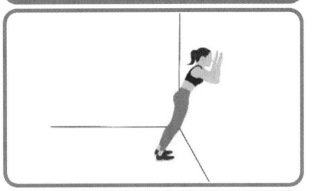

Page 16

LOWER BODY EXERCISES

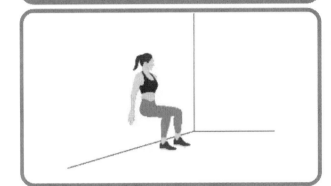

Page 26

UPPER BODY EXERCISES

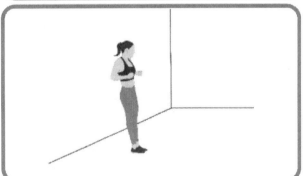

Page 38

TOTAL BODY EXERCISES

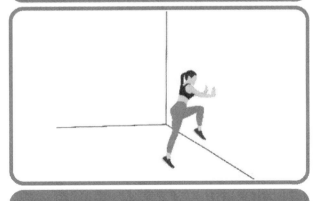

Page 50

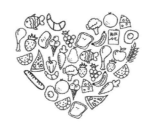

Your Free Gift

As a way of saying thanks for your purchase, I'm offering the **28-Days Diet Plan eBook for FREE** to my readers.

To get instant access just scan the QR code at the end of this book!

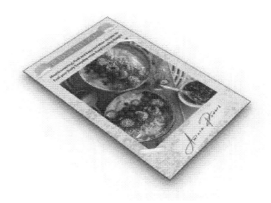

Here's what makes this journey truly amazing:

- **Plant-Powered Living:** I've designed this plan with a strong plant-based focus, providing you with all the nutrients you need while reducing your meat consumption;

- **Effortless Eats:** Life can get crazy, and we get it. These recipes are designed with your busy schedule in mind. You won't need to be a gourmet chef; these meals are quick and easy to prepare.

- **Speedy Deliciousness:** Time is precious, and I value yours. These recipes are efficient and, most importantly, delicious. You don't have to sacrifice taste for health;

- **Weekend Indulgence:** Weekends are for relaxing and enjoying life. I encourage you to treat yourself. Whether it's brunch with friends or a cozy night in with your favorite comfort food, it's all about balance.

If you're ready to supercharge your weight loss results and experience a transformation like never before, make sure to grab the free book.

YOUR TRANSFORMATION WITH WALL PILATES

Welcome to the world of Wall Pilates! In this journey we will embark on a fitness adventure that goes beyond traditional exercise routines and takes your body and mind to new heights. As a personal trainer and writer, my mission consists of empowering women through fitness.

I am excited to guide you through this incredible method of exercise that combines the principles of Pilates with the support of a wall. At its core, Wall Pilates is more than just physical strength and flexibility; it's a holistic approach that nurtures your mind, body, and spirit.

This unique training technique utilizes bodyweight exercises on a wall to enhance stability challenge your muscles and achieve better results. Whether you're starting as a beginner or an experienced enthusiast looking for a fresh approach, Wall Pilates will meet you where you are and motivate you to surpass your limits.

So why choose Wall Pilates? Because it's a game changer!

It sculpts and tones your body while boosting your confidence and can be practiced in the comfort of your home, improving posture and cultivating inner strength. Through carefully crafted exercises Wall Pilates engages core muscles, challenges balance and targets specific muscle groups for a leaner physique. But beyond physical changes Wall Pilates offers a transformative experience that empowers you inside and out.

In "Wall Pilates Workouts for Women" we'll explore various exercises designed to target different muscle groups, promote weight loss and sculpt your body.

Each exercise is thoroughly explained with step-by-step instructions and illustrations so you can safely perform them at home. The beauty of Wall Pilates lies in its accessibility; no fancy equipment or expensive gym memberships required: just you, a wall and the determination to transform your life.

The aim of this book is to motivate and inspire you on your unique journey. It is my hope that you will feel empowered and believe in your own strength as you embrace this transformative experience. Throughout the pages I will share personal insights, tips, and techniques to support you in maximizing your results and overcoming any challenges you may face.

It's important to remember that progress may not always be steady but every step forward is a victory in itself. In addition, there is a chapter dedicated to creating comprehensives 6-week workout plans designed to provide structure, variety, and progressive challenges according to your fitness level and goals.

Your transformation with Wall Pilates begins now!

Together we will break through barriers, go beyond limits and discover the incredible strength within you. Embrace the power of Wall Pilates and prepare yourself for the amazing changes that await you; let's embark on this empowering journey together as we unlock your full potential.

Remember, this is more than just a workout plan, it's a transformation.

Get ready to redefine what your body can do and embrace the best version of yourself.

Get ready to strengthen your abs, lift your booty and experience the exhilaration of Wall Pilates.

Are you prepared for this life changing journey? Let's begin!

1. INTRODUCTION TO WALL PILATES

In this chapter, we will explore the unique benefits of Wall Pilates, the essential equipment needed for home practice, and the importance of safety guidelines and proper posture.

THE UNIQUE BENEFITS OF WALL PILATES

Welcome to the world of Wall Pilates, where the fusion of Pilates principles and the support of a wall brings forth a multitude of unique benefits that set it apart from other exercise methods. In this section we will explore these distinct advantages that make Wall Pilates an exceptional fitness practice.

Firstly, Wall Pilates offers a holistic approach to fitness and well-being. Unlike many exercise modalities that focus solely on physical strength and aesthetics, Wall Pilates encompasses the mind, body and spirit.

It fosters a deep connection and balance within oneself that goes beyond the superficial. Through this practice you are empowered to develop not only physical strength and flexibility but also mental clarity. One exceptional benefit of Wall Pilates lies in its ability to provide enhanced stability and support.

The wall serves as a prop that assists in maintaining proper alignment during movements. This enables you to concentrate on executing exercises with precision and control. With this stability element, people of varying fitness levels can engage in Wall Pilates and reap its transformative effects.

Sculpting and toning the entire body is another remarkable advantage offered by Wall Pilates. By targeting specific muscle groups through controlled movements, you can achieve a lean and stunning physique.

Moreover, the focus on core strength improves posture and spinal alignment, reducing the risk of back pain or injuries. Wall Pilates also provides an opportunity for enhancing body awareness and proprioception: the perception of one's body position in space, as you perform exercises with wall support, you become more attuned to your movement nuances.

This heightened awareness allows for fine tuning technique deepening your mind body connection and cultivating greater control and grace in your daily activities. Additionally, by engaging multiple muscle groups simultaneously, Wall Pilates exercises promote functional fitness preparing your body for everyday life demands. They mimic real life movements such as coordination tasks or balancing challenges improving coordination skills, balance proficiency as well as flexibility. These benefits extend beyond the exercise studio enabling you to move with ease and confidence in your daily tasks and recreational pursuits.

Summarizing, Wall Pilates offers a unique and exceptional approach to fitness that goes beyond physical strength and aesthetics. With its holistic nature stability support sculpting potential, enhanced body awareness and functional fitness promotion this practice sets itself apart. Embark on the journey of Wall Pilates today to experience its transformative effects firsthand.

Wall Pilates offers not just physical benefits but also significantly impacts mental well-being. Immersed in the practice, attentively focusing on breath control as well as purposeful movement bestows upon oneself a mindful state along with tranquillity.

This meditative experience crafted through rhythmic flow during exercises of Wall Pilates fosters stress reduction, cultivates better concentration-and ultimately establishes overall well-being. This relatively low-impact however highly effective form of exercise triumphs being indulged by individuals across all age groups-with varied fitness levels. Eminently gentle on joints while still rendering an invigorating workout which elevates cardiovascular fitness, muscular endurance coupled with flexibility. In fact, this practice is capable of being adapted specifically for circumstances such as recuperating from injuries.

Quite noticeably, the empowerment to discover a reservoir of inner strength lies within the practice, transforming one's perspective propelling towards a journey of embracing resilience and acquiring positive mindsets.

An amalgamation enveloping one's consciousness, physicality as well as spirituality culminating into self-awareness, self-confidence and self-acceptance; in turn allowing for transformative personal growth- leading individuals towards fulfilling lives.

Be prepared to experience the profound enhancements Wall Pilates has in store as it uncovers your body, mind altogether your spirit's full potential together. Let's take on this empowering voyage exploring oneself manifesting stronger healthier, genuinely vibrant versions.

ESSENTIAL EQUIPMENT FOR HOME PRACTICE

Discover the joy of practicing Wall Pilates in the comfort of your own home with minimal equipment required! Wall Pilates offers a versatile exercise method that harnesses the support of a wall to enhance stability and engagement without relying on complex or costly gear. Now let's explore the essential items needed to establish a safe and effective home practice space tailored specifically for Wall Pilates. This begins with selecting an appropriate wall, choose one with enough space and clearance for comfortable execution of all exercises without restrictions.

Ensure there are no sharp edges or objects present that could potentially cause harm during practice sessions. Also vital is confirming that the wall is structurally sound enough to support your body weight throughout each exercise. To maximize comfort and support while performing floor exercises, its' highly recommended investing in a high-quality exercise mat.

The ideal mat will possess adequate thickness providing cushioning for the joints and spine allowing smooth execution of exercises with ease and comfort. Seek a mat with good grip to minimize slippage and one that's' easy to clean and maintain. As you progress in your Wall Pilates journey you might consider incorporating additional props or accessories to enhance your workouts.

These, however, are non-essential and optional for a successful home practice.

The main focus in Wall Pilates primarily lies in utilizing the wall and your own bodyweight for resistance and stability. Small hand weights or resistance bands can be introduced as props to intensify challenge and diversify workouts, they can effectively increase resistance while delivering additional strength training benefits.

Nevertheless, if you prefer simplicity or are just beginning your practice, remarkable results can be still achieved using just your bodyweight along with the support of the wall.

Stability balls can prove beneficial for exercises involving balance, coordination, and stability. In addition to equipment selection made dynamically during exercises, establishing an environment facilitating workouts becomes exceedingly crucial.

Going along this line, it becomes significant which practicing without disturbances needs consideration alongside pro-activeness toward cleaning, decluttering, and allowing proper ventilation. To enhance disposition conducive for exercise, incorporating soft background music or using essential oils can aid in establishing tranquillity.

As equipment becomes a crucial staple for Wall Pilates enthusiasts, uncomplicatedness is the defining characteristic. Translating this to perspective helps appreciate the simple yet adaptable allure of Wall Pilates. Regardless of whether an allocated home gym space or even a modest corner within the living room suffices, a setting that nurtures immersive opportunities is always achievable. Always mindful about safety and diligent regard to working out free from injury, having regular safety checks inspections on your wall & mat reassures functionality security.

If at any point you encounter any discomforts or acute pain signalling possible harm, adjust accordingly or in worst-case scenario, discontinue your activity entirely. Relying upon these core fundamental principles coupled with rightfully positioned equipment goals sets us ready for our journey into Wall Pilates at home; remember how Wall Pilates wonderfully empowers us through its elegance and accessibility without burdening ourselves with intricate equipment schemes. Call out to the unexplored possibilities while anchoring yourself into an endeavor cultivating strength, good health, and empowerment.

SAFETY GUIDELINES AND PROPER POSTURE

When participating in any type of exercise, prioritizing safety is a must. This holds true for Wall Pilates as it involves various movements that require proper alignment, technique, and body awareness.

In this section we will discuss important safety guidelines and offer advice on maintaining correct posture during your Wall Pilates practice. Above all else it is crucial to consult with your healthcare provider prior to starting a new exercise program especially if you have existing medical conditions or injuries.

As you begin your Wall Pilates practice it is important to start slowly and listen to your body. Allow yourself time to adjust to the exercises and gradually increase the intensity and duration of your workouts, pushing yourself too hard too quickly can result in injuries and setbacks.

Always respect the limits of your body and avoid overexertion.

Proper alignment and posture are key factors in maximizing the benefits of Wall Pilates exercises while preventing injuries. Please keep these fundamental principles in mind:

- **Engage Your Core:** During your practice of Wall Pilates, it is important to consistently maintain a strong and active engagement of your core. Visualize a corset encircling your waist, delicately pulling your navel inward towards your spine. By activating your core in this manner, you are able to enhance stability offer support to your lower back and enhance control over your entire body.

- **Align Your Spine:** Through each exercise performed, always prioritize preserving optimal spinal alignment with unwavering dedication. Envision an invisible thread delicately drawing upwards from above, gently extending and aligning every vertebrae in your backbone. Vigilance against both slouching and overextending of the lower back is vital in preventing undue stress upon the spine yielding potential discomfort. Keep striving towards maintaining neutrality within the positioning of all curves inherent within one's own individual spinal anatomy.

- **Protect Your Joints:** Please pay close attention to the alignment of your joints while performing the exercises. It is important to make sure that your knees are in line with your toes and to avoid excessive rolling of the ankles either inward or outward. Additionally, remember to maintain a gentle bend in your joints instead of locking them as this can lead to unnecessary stress on the joints.

- **Breathe Mindfully:** It is crucial to employ the appropriate breathing technique when engaging in Wall Pilates. Remember to synchronize your breath with your movements. Taking deep inhalations through your nostrils and complete exhalations through your mouth. By allowing your breath to direct the flow of each exercise, you will foster relaxation and ensure oxygenation of your muscles.

- **Modify When Needed:** It is important to listen to your body and make adjustments to exercises when needed. If you experience pain, discomfort or if an exercise feels too difficult it is completely acceptable to modify it or select a different exercise that is more suitable for your current level of fitness. Its' crucial to keep in mind that each person has a unique body. So, what may work for someone else may not necessarily work for you.

To further ensure your safety during Wall Pilates, follow these important guidelines:

1. **Warm-Up:** Before you begin your Wall Pilates practice it is advisable to warm up your body with some gentle movements. This will help improve circulation slightly raise your heart rate and properly prepare your muscles for the upcoming exercise. In the upcoming chapter, I will provide you some warm-up exercises to properly begin your workout session.

2. **Progress Gradually:** As you gain more confidence with the exercises you may progressively elevate both the intensity and complexity. Nevertheless, it is essential to always proceed at a pace that feels comfortable and within your capabilities. Hastening into advanced movements without properly mastering the foundational ones can heighten the likelihood of sustaining injuries.

3. **Stay Hydrated:** To optimize your performance during Wall Pilates practice it is crucial to prioritize your hydration. Remember to keep a water bottle within easy reach and take regular sips before during and after your session. This will help replenish fluids and ensure that you are at your best throughout the practice.

4. **Create a Safe Environment:** Please ensure that your practice area is free of any hazards or obstacles that may potentially lead to accidents. It is important to remove any sharp objects or tripping hazards from the area and ensure that you have enough space to move around without restrictions.

5. **Listen to Your Body:** Please make sure to be attentive to any indications of pain or discomfort while you engage in your practice. If you notice that something doesn't feel quite right take a moment to pause and evaluate the situation. It is crucial to distinguish between muscular fatigue and any pain that could potentially signify an injury. If you are uncertain, I highly recommend seeking guidance from a knowledgeable fitness professional.

For a secure and efficient Wall Pilates practice, it is essential to follow these safety guidelines diligently while maintaining proper posture throughout. Always bear in mind that your well-being should take precedence above all else; hence by giving utmost importance to safety measures, you can ensure optimal results from every workout session with minimized risks of harm or injury.

Now equipped with the necessary knowledge for ensuring personal welfare during this transformative experience known as Wall Pilates, let us proceed towards exploring specific exercises as well as techniques aimed at sculpting the body effectively along with improving overall posture; an opportunity for unlocking our truest potential within ourselves awaits! Embrace this journey with mindfulness and consciousness towards safety, and rest assured, the rewards will be both fulfilling and empowering.

2. WARM-UP AND STRETCHING

In this chapter, we will explore the essential components of warming up and stretching in preparation for your Wall Pilates practice A proper warm-up and stretching routine not only helps prevent injuries but also primes your body for optimal performance and flexibility. Within this chapter, we will delve into dynamic movements to prepare the body and various stretching techniques that will enhance your flexibility and range of motion.

DYNAMIC MOVEMENTS TO PREPARE THE BODY

Welcome to the invigorating world of dynamic movements that will prepare your body for the transformative Wall Pilates practice ahead. In this section, we will explore a variety of dynamic exercises designed to increase blood flow, activate your muscles, and slightly elevate your heart rate. These movements serve as an essential warm-up.

Awakening your body and mind for the challenges and rewards of your Wall Pilates workout, dynamic warm-up exercises are an integral part of any effective fitness routine. They not only improve circulation but also enhance joint mobility and muscular activation.

By engaging in dynamic movements, you initiate a shift from your everyday activities to a focused and energized state, priming your body for optimal performance. The beauty of dynamic warm-up exercises lies in their ability to replicate the movements and patterns encountered during your Wall Pilates practice.

By mimicking these motions, you activate relevant muscle groups, reinforce proper movement patterns, and improve overall coordination and stability. During the warm-up phase, you have the opportunity to connect with your body, heighten body awareness, and tune into the present moment; embrace the sensation of awakening muscles.

Gradually increasing heart rate and breath synchronizing with each movement, this mindful approach sets the tone for a transformative and empowering Wall Pilates experience.

Within this section, I will guide you through a series of dynamic movements, providing detailed instructions and illustrations to ensure proper execution. These exercises may include arm circles, leg swings, torso twists, and dynamic lunges. Each movement is carefully selected to activate major muscle groups while increasing flexibility and enhancing overall body readiness. As you engage in these dynamic movements, pay attention to fluid transitions and the quality of movement, emphasizing control, precision, and a full range of motion, allowing your body to explore its capabilities while maintaining proper alignment.

Bear in mind that this activity aims at preparing your body instead of depleting it. Should you feel any pain or discomfort while performing these exercises, it is crucial that you modify the movements or lower their intensity accordingly, as you remain in full control over your workout experience.

Incorporating dynamic movements into your pre-workout routine brings forth a myriad of benefits beyond mere physical readiness. It presents an opportunity to transition mentally into your workout session by leaving behind the stresses and distractions encountered throughout the day.

Gear all focus towards finding rhythm among movements while actively sensing muscle engagement; cultivating mindfulness and deep presence along this journey. Don't forget that stimulating exercises also lead one to experience a genuine outburst of energy which further adds excitement upon embarking on empowering Wall Pilates practice. Expect invigorating exercises as they awaken both potential locked within your physique and unleash primal fires within. It prepares you for what awaits throughout this transformative path confidently.

Hence, embrace such energetic movements as part of Wall Pilates practice, and you will surely enjoy these sudden surges coursing through your body; with awakening muscles growing stronger as anticipation continues building up. Imagine that this serves as an opportunity for revealing a radiant self, exceeding previously imposed limits, all accompanied by extraordinary strength that reveals a redefined version of self.

STRETCHING FOR IMPROVED FLEXIBILITY AND RANGE OF MOTION

Let's delve deeper into the fascinating world of stretching, an essential component of your pre workout routine that promotes improved flexibility and increased range of motion.

Effectively preparing them for the challenges and rewards that await you in your Wall Pilates practice, stretching not only benefits your physical performance but also plays a critical role in preventing injuries and aiding in post workout recovery. By incorporating stretching into your warm up routine, you can enhance your flexibility and reduce muscle tension, and optimize your body's ability to move freely and gracefully during your Wall Pilates workout. Stretching offers an opportunity to deeply connect with your body: cultivating mindfulness and embracing the present moment.

As you engage in these stretching exercises, concentrate on your breath, allowing it to guide your movements and deepen the connection between mind and body.

Embrace the invigorating sensation as your muscles gradually lengthen and let yourself relax into each stretch while maintaining a sense of ease and comfort. Within this section, I will comfortably guide you through a range of stretching exercises that specifically target major muscle groups.

Ultimately promoting flexibility and an increased range of motion, each exercise will be thoughtfully accompanied by detailed instructions and helpful illustrations to ensure that you maintain proper form and technique throughout.

Stretching exercises can be divided into two main categories: static stretching and dynamic stretching. Static stretching involves holding a stretch in a comfortable position for an extended period allowing the muscles to loosen up and elongate. On the other hand, dynamic stretching incorporates gentle yet controlled movements that gradually improve joint mobility.

Static stretches are particularly effective at releasing built up tension within the muscles as well as improving overall elasticity. Of course, dynamic stretching techniques focus on activating your muscles and preparing them for the dynamic movements encountered during your Wall Pilates practice.

Stretching provides a serene moment within your workout routine where self-care takes precedence. It serves as an opportunity for cultivating patience, self-compassion and appreciating what our bodies are capable of doing. Each stretch should be embraced as an act of self-love: a way showing respect for our bodies' unique needs and limitations.

Remember that flexibility is something that takes time, it is essential to maintain consistent practice in order to witness improvements in your range of motion and overall flexibility. Each stretching session should be approached with an open mind and curiosity allowing yourself to discover the incredible potential of your body for movement and adaptation. Incorporating stretching into your warm up routine not only enhances physical performance it also encourages the so called "mind-muscle connection" during Wall Pilates practice. It gives you an opportunity to tap into the full potential of your muscles by promoting proper alignment and enhancing body awareness throughout the workout. A better workout quality leads to better results.

As we progress through this book, don't forget to incorporate stretching exercises into your warm up routine before each Wall Pilates session. Take this chance to nurture your body, enrich flexibility and unlock new levels of freedom in movement. Stretching is a precious gift we give ourselves: a moment to honor and care for our bodies as we embark on this transformative Wall Pilates journey.

Are you ready for this exciting journey of stretching? Let's explore the techniques that will improve flexibility, increase range of motion and deepen mind body connection. Get ready to push past limits expand possibilities and experience the freedom that comes with having a flexible & mobile body.

FULL-BODY STRETCHING EXERCISES

In this section, we will explore several full body stretching exercises that aim to prepare your body for a rewarding Wall Pilates session.

These stretching exercises have been specifically designed to target major muscle groups improve flexibility and enhance your range of motion. Each exercise will be accompanied by detailed instructions to ensure you execute them correctly and obtain the maximum benefits from your stretching routine.

Static Stretches

Standing Forward Fold

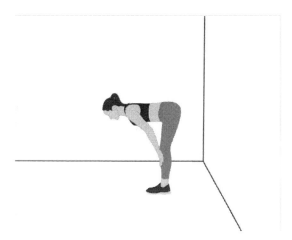

Assume an upright posture with your feet positioned hip width apart. Inhale deeply. Then gradually exhale while bending at the hips and lowering your upper body forward. Extending your hands towards the ground or placing them gently on your shins. Notice the sensation of stretching in your hamstrings, calves, and lower back. Maintain this position for a duration of 30 seconds to 1 minute as you continue to breathe deeply.

Chest Opener

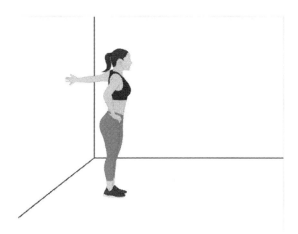

Stand a few inches away from a wall, maintaining an upright posture. Begin by extending one arm alongside your body and placing your palm flat against the wall at shoulder height. The fingers should be pointing behind you.

Slowly rotate your torso in the opposite direction from the extended arm, creating a gentle twist. You should feel a mild stretch in the chest and shoulder of the extended arm. Keep your core engaged and your hips facing forward.

Hold this position for 20-30 seconds, focusing on deep and controlled breaths. Allow your muscles to relax into the stretch, gradually increasing the intensity. After completing one side, switch to the other arm and repeat the stretch.

Quadriceps Stretch

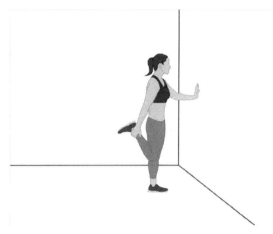

Stand up straight and use a wall for support. Begin by bending one knee and raising your heel towards your glutes. Then reach down and grasp your foot or ankle with the hand on the same side. You should feel a gentle stretch in the front of your thigh. Remember to maintain this position for 30 seconds to 1 minute on each side. Taking deep breaths throughout.

Spinal Twist

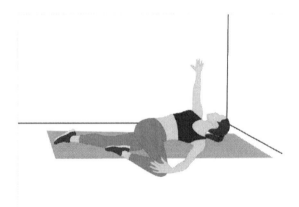

Assume a seated position on the floor. Extending your legs in front of you. Gradually bend your right knee and position your right foot outside of your left thigh. Rest your left elbow on the outer side of your right knee and gradually rotate your upper body to the right. Directing your gaze over your right shoulder. Notice the soothing sensation as you stretch your spine and hip region. Maintain this pose for approximately 30 seconds to 1 minute on both sides. Focusing on deep, controlled breaths throughout.

Child's Pose

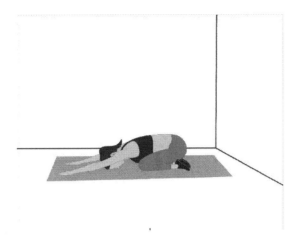

Assume a position on your hands and knees then gently ease yourself back onto your heels and gradually lower your forehead towards the mat. You may choose to extend your arms in front of you or opt to rest them comfortably alongside your body. Take a moment to embrace the exquisite sensation of stretching that encompasses your back, hips, and shoulders. Allow yourself to remain in this position for a duration of 1 to 2 minutes. All while inhaling and exhaling deeply with each breath you take.

Dynamic Stretches

Arm Circles

Assume a strong posture with your feet positioned hip width apart. Extend your arms out to the sides keeping them parallel to the ground. Initiate gentle circular movements with your arms gradually expanding the size of these circles as you go. Once you've completed several rotations alter the direction of the circles. Aim to sustain this exercise for a duration of 30 seconds to 1 minute. Ensuring that your movements remain steady and deliberate.

Leg Swings

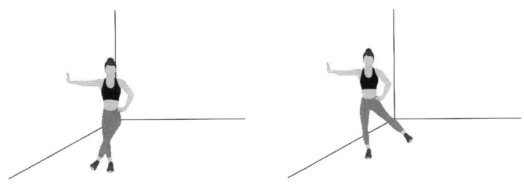

When starting out with this exercise, grant yourself sufficient balance by standing alongside a solid wall or supportive structure nearby that allows for stability throughout the activity duration. Begin by initiating gentle swings of one leg: swing it forward first followed by swinging it backward – ensure that the entire process keeps the leg naturally straightened at all times without giving way to unnecessary bending movements. To maximize effectiveness incrementally increase the amplitude of each swing, maintain this pattern for 10 to 15 swings prior to switching over and repeating the exercises with your other leg. While focusing on having mastery of precise, controlled movements, meticulously sense and appreciate a soothing extension in both your hamstring and hip flexor muscles.

Torso Twists

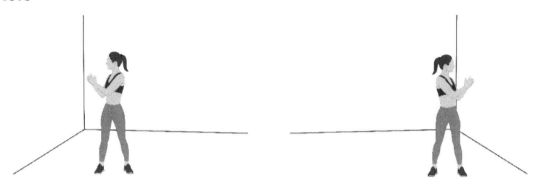

Stand with your feet shoulder width apart maintaining an upright posture. Choose whether to place your hands firmly on your hips or interlace your fingers behind your head. Gently pivot your upper body towards the right side and then to the left side. Ensuring that your hips align with the movement. Continue this rotation for a total of 10 to 15 twists. While actively engaging your core muscles and appreciating the pleasant stretch in both your obliques and lower back.

Walking Lunges with a Twist

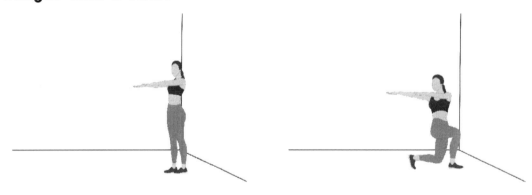

Take a step forward with your right foot. Assuming a lunge position. While lowering yourself into the lunge, kindly twist your upper body towards the right. Afterward gently push off with your right foot bringing both of your feet together, proceed to repeat the lunge and twist on the left side. By doing so you will experience a delightful stretch in your hips, quads, and obliques.

Ankle Circles

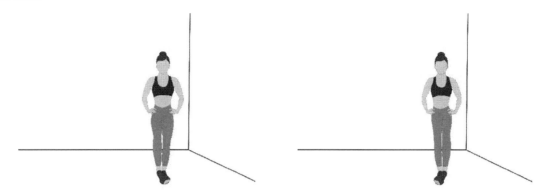

To perform this exercise, stand upright with your feet positioned hip width apart. Start by lifting one foot off the ground and gently rotate your ankle in circular motions. First in one direction and then in the opposite direction. Repeat this movement for a total of 10 to 15 circles before switching to the other foot. Keep your focus on maintaining a fluid and controlled motion throughout as you aim to feel a gentle stretch and enhance mobility in your ankles.

To maximize the productivity and enjoyment of your Wall Pilates sessions, it is wise to incorporate both static and dynamic stretching exercises into your warm up routine.

These specific stretches meticulously target key muscle groups, effectively preparing them for the physical demands associated with your practice while simultaneously enhancing overall flexibility and range of joint motion. Continually integrating these stretching exercises into your pre workout routine as we progress through this book would be highly advantageous.

By doing so, you will reap remarkable benefits including improved flexibility, increased mobility as well as an enriched mind body connection. Each stretch carried out during warm up represents an act of self-care toward nurturing your own physique while concurrently building a strong foundation for a transformative Wall Pilates experience.

Get ready to embark upon this profound voyage towards attaining superior levels of flexibility balanced alongside elegance and strength in every aspect, both mentally and physically. Allow these full body stretches to unlock your body's potential ignite a fervent enthusiasm within and steadily guide you towards the exceptional advantages that manifest as a result of engaging in Wall Pilates.

3. CORE AND ABDOMINAL EXERCISES

This chapter is dedicated entirely to helping you strengthen and carve out a well-toned midsection through an assortment of core and abdominal exercises. A strong core holds importance not just for its appealing appearance but also due to its contribution towards overall stability, proper posture maintenance as well as facilitating functional movement.

Within these pages lies valuable information about various exercises meticulously designed to target different areas within your core including the rectus abdominis; obliques; and deeper stabilizing muscles. Inclusion of such exercises in your routine brings about challenges while improving both strength in the core region along with boosting muscular endurance whilst reinforcing control over abdominal movements.

WALL PLANK FOR CORE ACTIVATION AND STABILITY

When it comes to honing a powerful set of core muscles concentrating on areas like your abdominals, back, and glutes few exercises prove more effective than engaging in wall planks. The benefits extend beyond basic strength-training as they enhance overall steadiness while fostering improved posture throughout their execution process. The comprehensive approach here aims not only at acquainting you with each step but also at providing valuable professional advice on correct-form implementation resulting in optimal results desired.

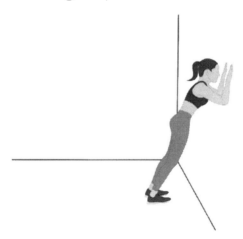

Step-by-Step Guide

1. Start by standing facing a wall, approximately arms-length away. Place your palms flat against the wall, shoulder-width apart and at chest level.

2. Step back with both feet, maintaining a hip-width distance between them. Your body should form a straight line from your head to your heels.

3. Engage your core muscles by drawing your navel towards your spine. This will create a strong foundation for the exercise.

4. Keep your neck and spine aligned by looking at the floor slightly in front of you, maintaining a neutral head position.

5. Distribute your weight evenly between your hands and feet, ensuring stability and balance throughout the exercise.

Tips

- Focus on maintaining a strong and stable core throughout the entire duration of the exercise.

- Keep your shoulders relaxed and away from your ears. Avoid shrugging or tensing the upper traps.

- Engage your glutes and legs by squeezing your buttocks and gently pressing your heels into the ground. This will help to activate the posterior chain and maintain proper alignment.

- Breathe deeply and consistently throughout the exercise. Inhale through your nose and exhale through your mouth, allowing your breath to fuel your movements and promote relaxation.

- If you feel discomfort or strain in your wrists, try modifying the exercise by performing the wall plank on your forearms instead of your palms. This will alleviate pressure on the wrists while still engaging the core muscles effectively.

Progression

Once you have mastered the basic wall plank, you can challenge yourself by incorporating variations and progressions to further strengthen your core and improve stability. Here are a few options you can try:

- **Extended Arm Plank:** Instead of placing your palms flat against the wall at shoulder height, extend your arms fully, resting your hands on the wall above your head. This will increase the demands on your core and upper body.

- **One-Leg Wall Plank:** Lift one foot off the ground and hold the wall plank position with only one foot supporting your body weight. Alternate between legs to work both sides evenly. This variation adds an extra stability challenge and engages the muscles in your standing leg.

- **Wall Side Plank:** Begin in the wall plank position, then rotate your body to the side, resting on one hand and stacking your feet. Hold this side plank position, engaging your obliques and lateral core muscles. Repeat on both sides for balanced strength development.

Bear in mind that consistency is key if you wish to reap the rewards brought about by engaging regularly in wall plank exercises. Gradually work towards integrating this exercise into your standard workout routine steadily increasing both its duration and difficulty level as time progresses alongside improvements made to your core strength. Display patience, dedication, and an unwavering commitment to proper form as these are essential elements required for achieving a stable and robust core utilizing the power of wall planks.

Rest easy knowing that not only will these exercises provide support during various daily activities but they will also augment the benefits derived from practicing Wall Pilates too. Embrace the challenges imposed by this exercise routine whilst simultaneously embracing the transformations it can bring about within your core strength itself. During each session take a moment to visualize precisely how hard at work your core muscles truly are as they assist you with every breath taken and movement executed. Experience firsthand the feelings evoked by stability, strength, and sheer power radiating outward from deep within, qualities which shall serve to embolden any efforts undertaken throughout one's personal fitness journey.

WALL LEG RAISES FOR LOWER ABS AND HIP FLEXOR STRENGTH

Are you ready to sculpt and strengthen your lower abs and hip flexors? Look no further than the powerful and effective wall leg raises exercise. This particular exercise is designed to target specific muscle groups in your core ultimately helping you achieve a toned and defined midsection.

In this section, I will provide you with a detailed guide on how to correctly execute wall leg raises, as well as emphasize their incredible aesthetic benefits. Additionally, I'll offer you valuable tips that can help you maximize your results when it comes to achieving a flat and toned stomach it is crucial to focus on the lower abs and hip flexors. Thankfully the wall leg raises exercise allows you to specifically engage these muscle groups, facilitating the creation of the sculpted midsection you desire. By incorporating wall leg raises into your routine you can effectively strengthen your core muscles while also improving stability and posture.

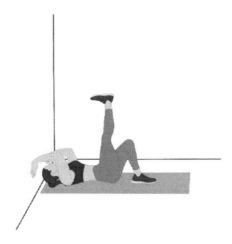

Step-by-Step Guide

1. Begin by lying on the floor face up, with your head close to the wall. Place your palms flat against the wall, maintaining a shoulder-width distance between them.

2. Apply a light pressure with the palms of your hands on the wall to maintain good stability, supporting your upper body.

3. Engage your core muscles by drawing your navel towards your spine. This will create a strong foundation for the exercise and ensure proper alignment.

4. Slowly lift one leg straight out in front of you, until it is perpendicular to the ground. Avoid arching your back or compensating with momentum.

5. With control, lower your leg back down towards the ground, maintaining a slight bend in your knee. Ensure a smooth and controlled movement throughout the exercise.

6. Repeat the movement with the opposite leg, alternating between legs for a balanced workout.

Tips

- Focus on the quality of each repetition rather than the quantity. Performing slow and controlled leg raises will maximize the engagement of your lower abs and hip flexors.

- Keep your core muscles activated throughout the exercise to maintain stability and prevent any excessive arching or rounding of the back.

- Maintain a relaxed and neutral upper body position, avoiding unnecessary tension in your shoulders, neck, and jaw.

- Breathe steadily throughout the exercise, inhaling through your nose and exhaling through your mouth. This will promote relaxation and enhance your mind-body connection.

- If you feel discomfort or strain in your lower back, you may need to reduce the range of motion or modify the exercise by performing smaller leg raises. Always listen to your body and adjust accordingly.

Progression

As you become more comfortable with wall leg raises, you can challenge yourself by incorporating variations and progressions to further enhance your lower abs and hip flexor strength. Here are a few options to consider:

- **Knee-to-Chest Wall Raises:** Instead of lifting your leg straight out in front of you, bring your knee towards your chest, engaging your lower abs and hip flexors. Alternate between legs to work both sides evenly.

- **Paused Leg Raises:** after each repetition, when your leg returns to the starting position (hovering it just above the floor, without touching it), hold the position for 5 seconds. This variation introduces an isometric work on your core, iliac psoas and quadriceps, adding toughness to your workout.

Incorporating wall leg raises into your fitness routine consistently yields remarkable improvements in lower abdominal strength as well as hip flexor strength. Strengthening these muscles helps sculpt an impressive midsection that radiates self-assurance alongside vitality, virtues worth embracing wholeheartedly! Envision extraordinary results stimulated by each leg raise, picturing stronger lower abs along with enhanced tone in those hip flexors is essential.

Feel empowered while confidently dedicating yourself towards shaping your midsection, a personal transformation imbued with both satisfaction as well as pride awaits! Commitment drives success toward achieving such greatness; consistent determination is key during this rejuvenating process towards attaining a beautifully-sculpted core.

Remember: emphasis lies on preserving proper form while attentively considering what works best for your body's needs; thus prioritizing these aspects bolsters endurance whilst avoiding potential injuries. Encountering this exercise, never hesitate to foster enthusiasm, determination, and a tremendous sense of joy.

Please commemorate every accomplishment no matter how small it may seem! Acknowledging the progress made along one's journey reassures the importance of discipline while inspiring perseverance. Remember, transformation is within your grasp; allow wall leg raises to play an influential role throughout this admirable quest of yours. Let us embark on this journey united, embracing both strength and the intrinsic beauty that resides within you.

WALL ROLL-UPS FOR ABDOMINAL CONTROL AND FLEXIBILITY

Are you ready to tap into the potential of your core muscles and achieve a lean and sculpted midsection? Look no further than the dynamic yet simple exercise called Wall Roll-Ups. This exercise specifically targets your abdominal muscles. Boosting both their strength and flexibility.

I will provide you with detailed instructions and professional tips on how to properly perform Wall Roll-Ups, ensuring that you can attain optimal results.

If you strive for a well-defined and flexible core that is sure to catch attention wall roll ups serve as your secret weapon. This exercise actively engages all areas of your abdominal region, including the rectus abdominis, obliques, and deeper stabilizing muscles. By incorporating wall roll ups into your fitness routine, not only will you be able to develop a stronger midsection but also enhance overall flexibility levels.

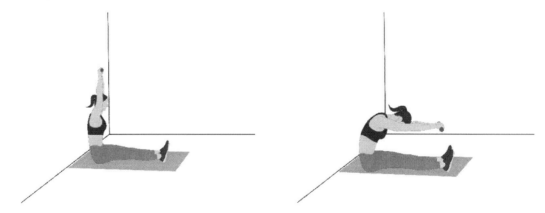

Step-by-Step Guide

1. Start by sitting on the floor with your back against the wall and your knees bent. Place your feet flat on the floor, hip-width apart.

2. Extend your arms straight out in front of you, parallel to the floor, with your palms facing down.

3. Engage your core by drawing your navel towards your spine. This will create a stable and strong foundation for the exercise.

4. Slowly begin to roll your spine off the wall, one vertebra at a time, until your body is in a C-curve position, with your shoulder blades lifted off the wall. Your arms should still be extended in front of you.

5. Hold the C-curve position for a moment, engaging your abdominal muscles and feeling the stretch along your spine. Squeeze your core muscles as hard as you can.

6. Slowly roll your spine back down onto the wall, one vertebra at a time, until you return to the starting position.

Tips

- Focus on maintaining control and a slow, controlled movement throughout the exercise. Avoid using momentum to roll up and down.

- Keep your shoulders relaxed and away from your ears. Avoid tension in the neck and jaw.

- Breathe deeply and exhale as you roll up, engaging your core muscles. Inhale as you roll back down, maintaining a steady breath pattern.

- If you find it challenging to roll up, you can modify the exercise by placing your hands behind your thighs for additional support. As your strength improves, gradually reduce the assistance from your hands.

- Maintain a slight engagement of your lower abdominals throughout the entire exercise to protect your lower back and enhance core activation.

Progression

As you develop a stronger familiarity with wall roll ups, you have the opportunity to push yourself by incorporating different variations and progressions. These techniques will not only enhance their abdominal control and flexibility but also provide a new level of challenge. Here's an option to consider:

- **Side-to-Side Wall Roll-Ups:** Perform the roll-up as usual, but when you reach the top position, rotate your torso to one side and touch the opposite hand to the opposite leg. Return to the center, then rotate to the other side. This variation targets the obliques and adds a rotational element to the exercise.

By consistently incorporating Wall Roll-Ups into your fitness routine incredible aesthetic benefits await. Your abdominal muscles will strengthen and become more defined while simultaneously experiencing improved flexibility with an increased range of motion. Visualize your desired beautifully sculpted midsection as you partake in this exercise envisioning how tight and toned your core is becoming.

With each repetition consciously observe how hard your abdominal muscles are working, tightening and toning with every roll up performed. Experience heightened empowerment and confidence through the development of a strong and agile core. As a personal trainer dedicated to guiding you on this path towards self-improvement, I am here to support every step of the way. Together, let's unleash the full potential of your core and achieve the body you've always dreamed of!

WALL SIDE CRUNCHES FOR OBLIQUE SCULPTING

Would you like to achieve well defined and sculpted oblique muscles that will enhance your waistline and create an eye-catching hourglass figure? Here you are the powerful exercise called Wall Side Crunches. This exercise specifically targets the oblique muscles helping you achieve a sleek and toned midsection.

We are going through the execution of Wall Side Crunches, providing clear instructions and professional tips to help you maximize your results. If you are looking to have a slim waistline and a beautifully sculpted midsection, incorporating Wall Side Crunches into your fitness routine can be a game changer. This exercise focuses on your oblique muscles, which are located along the sides of your torso. By targeting these muscles, you can create a tapered waistline, enhance overall body symmetry and achieve an aesthetically pleasing physique.

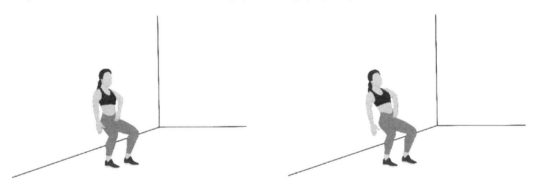

Step-by-Step Guide

1. Start by standing next to a wall with your feet shoulder-width apart and your arm closest to the wall extended overhead, resting against the wall for support.

2. Position your body so that your arm is slightly above shoulder height, and your feet are a comfortable distance away from the wall (your knees should be bent at 90 degrees angle).

3. Engage your core by drawing your navel towards your spine. This will create a strong foundation for the exercise and ensure proper alignment.

4. Slowly lean sideways towards the wall, bending at the waist and keeping your upper body aligned. Imagine bringing your shoulder down towards your hip.

5. As you lean towards the wall, focus on contracting your oblique muscles on the opposite side. Feel the side crunch as you engage your obliques to lift your torso back up to a neutral position.

6. Repeat the movement for the desired number of repetitions on one side, then switch to the other side.

Tips

- Maintain control throughout the exercise by performing the movement slowly and deliberately. Avoid any jerking or swinging motions.

- Focus on the quality of the contraction in your oblique muscles. Squeeze and engage them as you perform the side crunch, emphasizing the mind-muscle connection.

- Keep your shoulders relaxed and away from your ears. Imagine lengthening your neck and maintaining a proud posture throughout the exercise.

- Breathe naturally and exhale as you perform the side crunch. Inhale as you return to the starting position.

- If you find it challenging to maintain balance, place your hand against the wall for additional support. This will help you stabilize and focus on targeting your obliques.

Progression

As you become more comfortable with regular Wall Side Crunches, you can challenge yourself by incorporating variations and progressions to further sculpt and strengthen your oblique muscles. Here are a few options to consider:

- **Weighted Wall Side Crunches:** Hold a dumbbell or a weighted object against your side as you perform the side crunches. The added resistance will increase the intensity and further engage your oblique muscles.

- **Dynamic Side Plank Crunches:** From a side plank position against the wall, lower your hips towards the ground, then use your oblique muscles to lift your hips back up to the starting position. This variation combines the benefits of a side plank and a side crunch, providing a full-body challenge.

- **Alternating Side Crunches:** Instead of performing consecutive side crunches on one side, alternate between sides for each repetition. This variation adds variety and symmetry to your workout.

By integrating wall side crunches into your fitness routine consistently remarkable aesthetic advantages will become evident. Strengthening and defining your oblique muscles will lead to a slender waistline and an admirable hourglass figure. Envision the exquisitely sculpted midsection you desire, allowing the endeavor towards a toned waistline to inspire and spur you forward.

Embrace this challenge and strive for new accomplishments with each side crunch; experience the extraordinary might and vigor in your oblique muscles as they engage during the exercise and commemorate each repetition as progress towards your ultimate aspiration. Together, let us unlock the full capabilities of your oblique muscles and transform your midsection into a masterpiece!

WALL BICYCLE CRUNCHES FOR TOTAL CORE ENGAGEMENT

Are you prepared to take your core workout to the next level and achieve a sculpted strong midsection that catches attention? Well, I present you the dynamic and highly effective exercise known as Wall Bicycle Crunches.

This exercise engages several core muscles simultaneously providing complete core engagement and aiding in the accomplishment of a well-defined and toned midsection. If you aspire to possess a lean and sculpted midsection that radiates strength and confidence Wall Bicycle Crunches are the key to unlocking your cores full potential. This exercise focuses on multiple muscles in your core, including the rectus abdominis, obliques, and transverse abdominis.

By incorporating Wall Bicycle Crunches into your routine, you can strengthen and tone your entire midsection revealing the aesthetic benefits you've been striving for.

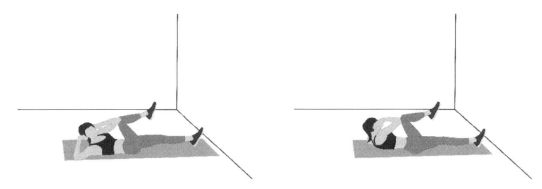

Step-by-Step Guide

1. Start by lying on your back. Place your hands lightly behind your head, elbows wide apart, and engage your core by drawing your navel towards your spine.

2. Lift your feet off the, creating a 90-degree angle with your knees. This will be your starting position.

3. Begin the movement by simultaneously bringing your right elbow towards your left knee while extending your right leg straight out, parallel to the ground.

4. As you complete the movement, switch sides, bringing your left elbow towards your right knee while extending your left leg straight out.

5. Continue alternating sides in a fluid and controlled motion, creating a pedaling or cycling motion with your legs, while twisting your torso to engage the obliques.

Tips

- Focus on the quality of each repetition rather than the speed. Perform the exercise in a controlled manner to engage and activate your core muscles effectively.

- Keep your elbows wide apart and avoid pulling on your neck during the movement. Your hands should gently support your head, allowing your core to do the work.

- Maintain a stable and engaged core throughout the exercise by avoiding excessive arching or rounding of your back.

- Breathe naturally and exhale as you bring your elbow towards your knee, focusing on engaging your core. Inhale as you switch sides and extend your leg.

- Visualize your core muscles contracting and working with each repetition. Feel the burn and embrace the challenge as you pedal through the movement.

Progression

As you enhance your skill in Wall Bicycle Crunches, it becomes possible to challenge yourself even more by integrating diverse variations and progressions that will intensify the engagement and fortify your core muscles. Consider the following options:

- **Bicycle Crunches with Extended Legs:** Instead of keeping your knees at a 90-degree angle, extend your legs fully, hovering them just above the ground. This variation increases the intensity and engages your core muscles even more.
- **Weighted Bicycle Crunches:** Hold a dumbbell or a weighted object (like small water bottles) in your hands as you perform the bicycle crunches. The added resistance challenges your core muscles further and helps promote strength and definition.
- **Slow and Controlled Bicycle Crunches:** Perform the bicycle crunches at a slower pace, focusing on the contraction and engagement of your core muscles throughout the entire range of motion. This variation emphasizes muscular control and endurance.

If you incorporate Wall Bicycle Crunches regularly into your fitness routine you will observe notable aesthetic benefits. Your core will grow stronger, more defined, and better prepared to support you during various activities and movements. It is important to embrace this process and envision obtaining the beautifully sculpted midsection that you desire.

With each repetition feel the power and strength radiate from your core as you pedal through them. Always remember to listen to your body respect its limits and gradually increase the intensity and difficulty of these exercises as you progress. Your core serves as an influential center of strength with wall bicycle crunches serving as a key element in unlocking its complete potential; together let us embark on this journey towards achieving the core of your dreams!

4. LOWER BODY EXERCISES

I am honored to introduce you to the exhilarating realm of lower body exercises! (I know, probably they're your favourite).

This chapter presents an assortment of remarkable wall-based exercises meticulously designed with the aim of fortifying your leg and tone up glute muscles, enhancing your balance and elevating overall lower body strength.

And of course, last but not least, achieving a juicy booty!

Brace yourself for an unparalleled transformation as I guide you towards sculpting and contouring your lower body in ways previously unexplored! Let us delve into this chapter together and uncover the remarkable exercises that lie ahead.

WALL SQUATS FOR LEG AND GLUTE STRENGTH

Are you ready to transform your legs and sculpt your glutes into beautiful works of art? Look no further than the powerful and effective exercise known as Wall Squats, the king of all lower body exercises. This exercise targets your quadriceps, hamstrings, and glutes, helping you build lower body strength and achieve a toned and shapely appearance.

If you desire strong toned legs and a firm lifted booty, Wall Squats are the perfect secret weapon for you. This exercise engages all your lower body muscles, promoting overall lower body strength and definition. Let's see how by incorporating Wall Squats into your routine, you can finally achieve the sculpted legs and toned glutes that have always been on your wishlist!

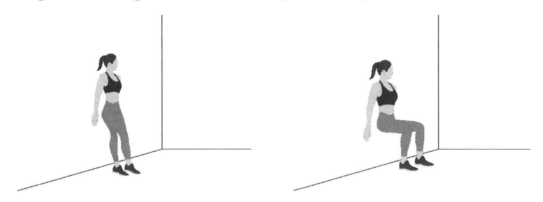

Step-by-Step Guide

1. Begin by standing with your back against a wall, ensuring that your feet are hip-width apart and positioned slightly away from the wall.

2. Slowly slide your back down the wall, bending your knees and lowering your body into a squat position. Your thighs should be parallel to the ground, and your knees should be directly above your ankles.

3. Keep your feet flat on the ground, pressing evenly through the heels and maintaining a neutral spine.

4. Engage your core by drawing your navel towards your spine, and maintain a proud posture throughout the exercise.

5. Hold the squat position for a desired amount of time or as long as you can maintain proper form and comfort.

6. To return to the starting position, push through your heels and straighten your legs, gradually sliding your back up the wall.

Tips

- Focus on proper form and alignment throughout the exercise. Keep your knees in line with your ankles, and avoid letting them collapse inward or extend past your toes.

- Engage your glutes and core muscles as you lower into the squat position. This will help stabilize your body and maximize the engagement of your lower body muscles.

- Breathe naturally and exhale as you lower into the squat. Inhale as you return to the starting position.

- As you descend into the squat, imagine sitting back into an imaginary chair, shifting your weight into your heels and maintaining a strong and balanced posture.

- Gradually increase the duration of your wall squats as your strength improves. Aim for 30 seconds to 1 minute initially and work your way up to longer holds or multiple sets.

Progression

Once you have mastered the basic Wall Squat, embarking on incorporating different variations and progressions can present a stimulating challenge to further augment the power of your legs and glutes. Considering upon these options might prove beneficial:

- **Weighted Wall Squats:** Hold a dumbbell or a weighted object against your chest or at your sides as you perform the wall squats. The added resistance increases the intensity and further engages your leg and glute muscles. As an overload, you can also use a resistance band fixing it under your feet.

- **One-Legged Wall Squats:** Perform the wall squats while balancing on one leg. This variation targets each leg individually, challenges your balance, and dramatically increases the demand on your muscles.

- **Wall Squat Pulses:** Instead of holding the squat position, perform small, controlled pulses up and down within the squat range. This variation adds a dynamic element and intensifies the muscle engagement. This is an excellent variation to feel a good pump in your glutes!

By incorporating Wall Squats consistently into your fitness routine, you will witness remarkable aesthetic benefits that are sure to delight! Prepare yourself for stronger quadriceps resulting in a more defined appearance!

Your hamstrings will also be beautifully toned while simultaneously lifting those glutes into their rightful place atop sculpted muscles! Visualize legs growing ever leaner yet increasingly powerful after each squat experience. Fully embrace this challenge while feeling those amazing sensations of endurance that ultimately lead toward achieving desired transformations of both leg glory and skyrocketing glute achievements!

Remember dear friend, progress requires intentional amounts of patience plus maintaining consistency throughout what can sometimes feel like an arduous process! Remember first things first… Start at an appropriate level which both challenges and allows for the correct form. Take time to genuinely connect with your body's limits and nourish it with the respect it deserves throughout this ever-increasingly intense challenge. Strive to incrementally increase intensity and difficulty of the exercises only as you observe progress in your journey! As always, remember I am here to encourage you at each step along this path to greatness! Approach these invigorating Wall Squats infused with unwavering determination, fueled by an unyielding confidence plus a belief deeply rooted within YOUR unique potential for monumental achievement!

Together let us embark on this epic adventure, bent on revealing both the quiet strength and stunning beauty which lies hidden within that oh-so-special lower body region of yours! Visualize waves of power plus astounding steadfastness radiating intensely from those amazing muscles engaged during each squat experience worthy of utter reverence & admiration!

WALL LUNGES FOR BALANCE AND LOWER BODY TONING

Here I am to present you Wall Lunges: an amazing exercise that focuses on targeting quadriceps, hamstrings, glutes, and calves for beautifully defined legs and a more powerful lower body with improved alignment.

In this section I present a detailed guide that will help you execute Wall Lunges efficiently. Alongside showcasing their incredible aesthetic benefits, I also provide valuable tips to help you achieve maximum results.

Utilizing the support of a wall during this exercise allows you to maintain proper form and balance while simultaneously engaging multiple muscle groups for an enhanced lower body workout experience. The advantages of incorporating Wall Lunges extend beyond toning or shaping; they contribute towards improving overall functional fitness through enhanced balance and stability, qualities that prove invaluable in everyday activities.

Prepare yourself to unlock the full potential of your lower body through the transformative power offered by Wall Lunges!

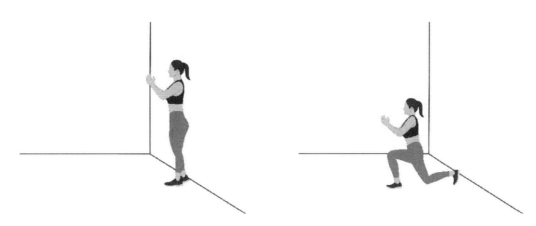

Step-by-Step Guide

1. Start by standing with your back against a wall and your feet hip-width apart, about a stride's distance away from the wall.

2. Place your hands on your hips or extend them in front of you for balance.

3. Take a step forward with your right foot, ensuring that your knee is directly above your ankle and your thigh is parallel to the ground. Your back heel should be lifted.

4. Slowly lower your body by bending both knees until your front thigh is parallel to the ground, and your back knee is hovering just above the floor. Keep your upper body upright and maintain a proud posture.

5. Push through your front heel to return to the starting position, engaging your leg muscles throughout the movement.

6. Repeat the lunge on the other side by stepping forward with your left foot and following the same movement pattern.

Tips

- Maintain proper form and alignment throughout the exercise. Keep your front knee in line with your ankle, and avoid letting it extend past your toes. Your back knee should be positioned slightly underneath your hip.

- Engage your core and focus on stability as you perform the lunges. This will help maintain balance and activate your deep core muscles.

- Keep your upper body tall and avoid leaning forward. Imagine a string pulling you up from the crown of your head.

- Breathe naturally throughout the movement, exhaling as you lower into the lunge and inhaling as you return to the starting position.

- Control your movements and avoid rushing through the exercise. Focus on the mind-muscle connection, feeling the work happening in your lower body muscles with each lunge.

- Gradually increase the depth of your lunges as your strength and flexibility improve. Aim to lower your front thigh parallel to the ground, but only go as far as your comfort and range of motion allow.

Progression

Once you have mastered the basic Wall Lunges, you can challenge yourself by incorporating variations and progressions to further enhance your lower body strength and stability. Here are a few options to consider:

- **Weighted Wall Lunges:** Hold a dumbbell or a weighted object in each hand as you perform the lunges. The added resistance will increase the intensity and further engage your leg muscles.

- **Lateral Wall Lunges:** Instead of stepping forward, step to the side, performing a lunge motion. This variation targets your inner and outer thighs, providing additional toning and sculpting benefits.

- **Plyometric Wall Lunges:** Add an explosive jump into your lunges, switching legs mid-air and landing softly into the next lunge. This variation adds a cardiovascular element and greatly increases the overall intensity of the exercise.

Witness incredible aesthetic benefits by consistently incorporating Wall Lunges into your fitness routine. Not only will this result in stronger, leaner, and more defined legs but also an improved balance and stability overall. Picture yourself confidently striding forward with each lunge feeling the power and strength from within your lower body. Embrace the challenge presented by these lunges; push past what you believed were limitations because their transformative capability for shaping your lower body is unparalleled.

It is important to remember that progress is a journey necessitating dedication, patience, along with consistency throughout. Be attentive to what your body communicates; respect its limits while gradually increasing the intensity and difficulty of the exercise as progress is achieved.

I encourage you to approach Wall Lunges with determination whilst maintaining focus on achieving remarkable results. So let's go further on this empowering journey where we uncover the hidden strength and beauty within our lower bodies.

With every lunge performed imagine how seamlessly muscles work together sculpting and toning our legs, recognize that you possess tremendous power capable of shaping and strengthening your lower body with Wall Lunges serving as the guiding force!

WALL BRIDGE FOR GLUTE ACTIVATION AND HAMSTRING STRENGTH

If you're eager to activate and shape your glute muscles while simultaneously strengthening your hamstrings, believe me, the astounding Wall Bridge exercise is a game changer. This remarkable exercise specifically targets both these muscle groups allowing individuals to attain a firmer buttocks appearance along with more defined leg muscles.

In this section, we will unveil an extensive yet professional guide on executing this highly effective exercise correctly while emphasizing its outstanding aesthetic benefits. Additionally, we'll cover valuable tips that will enable you to optimize your results when incorporating the Wall Bridge into your routine workouts.

The Wall Bridge stands as a powerful tool in enhancing lower body strength through activating ones' glute muscles alongside their hamstring counterparts purposefully. By leveraging a wall for support during this targeted workout modality proper posture maintenance becomes achievable along with proper muscle engagement leading to desired outcomes on the physical well-being front.

Regardless of the goal, lifted and sculpted glutes or amplified lower body strength, the utilization of the Wall Bridge remains a top-tier choice. Prepare yourself to unlock your glutes and hamstrings' true potential with this exceptional exercise. Let's pump your booty up!

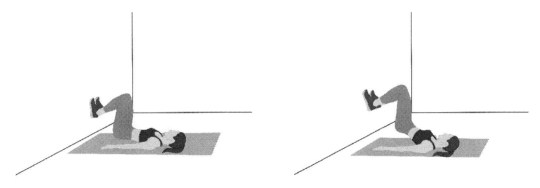

Step-by-Step Guide

1. Begin by lying on your back with your feet on the wall, hip-width apart. Your knees should be bent at approximately a 90-degree angle or slightly less.
2. Place your arms by your sides, palms facing down, for stability.
3. Press your feet firmly into the wall and engage your core by drawing your navel towards your spine.
4. Slowly lift your hips off the ground, driving through your heels, until your body forms a straight line from your knees to your shoulders.
5. Pause for a moment at the top, squeezing your glutes and engaging your hamstrings.
6. Lower your hips back down to the starting position with control, ensuring that your upper back remains in contact with the ground throughout the movement.

Tips

- Focus on proper form and alignment during the wall bridge exercise. Keep your feet flat on the wall, press through your heels, and avoid letting your knees collapse inward or extend beyond your toes.

- Engage your glutes and hamstrings as you lift your hips, ensuring that these muscles are doing the majority of the work. Visualize them contracting and working with each repetition.

- Avoid overarching your lower back or allowing your shoulders to shrug. Maintain a neutral spine and keep your shoulder blades gently pressed into the ground.

- Breathe naturally throughout the exercise, exhaling as you lift your hips and inhaling as you lower them.

- Gradually increase the duration of your wall bridge holds as your strength improves. Aim for 10-20 seconds initially and work your way up to longer holds or multiple sets.

Progression

After acquiring proficiency in the fundamental Wall Bridge exercise, you can elevate your skill level by introducing modifications and advancements that will amplify the effectiveness of targeting your glute and hamstring muscles. Below are several alternatives you may want to try:

- **Single-Leg Wall Bridge:** Lift one leg off the ground and perform the bridge with the opposite leg, focusing on maintaining stability and engaging your glutes and hamstrings unilaterally.

- **Resistance Band Wall Bridge:** Place a resistance band just above your knees and perform the bridge, actively pushing against the band to engage your glutes even more.

- **Marching Wall Bridge:** While holding the bridge position, alternate lifting your knees towards your chest, as if marching in place. This variation adds an extra challenge to your core stability and engages your hip flexors.

By consistently including Wall Bridges in your fitness routine, mind-blowing aesthetic benefits await you. Witness how your glutes become firmer, lifted, more defined; see how stronger & sculpted those hamstrings become!

Imagine envisioning your own booty turning into your best asset! Moreover, conquer challenges as they lead towards desired results achieved step by step. In doing so never forget listening intently attentively (even respectfully) both body & limits. Additionally, gradually increase intensity plus difficulty while progressing on path set forth.

Remember: any single "bridge" serves as chance not only connecting but strengthening simultaneously those all-wondrous-glutes-&-hammies! Embrace awesome burn, even embrace journey perceived! Lastly let the almighty power of said Wall Bridges transform you into an even stronger self, reaching heights otherwise unknown or thought unachievable! Proud personal trainer here, utterly encouraging to approach this wondrous task with utmost focus, determination and perhaps last by not least; belief in yourself that remarkable results can shall & will be achieved.

Unlock that long-hidden inner strength plus beauty inherent in available gluteus and hamstrings, forging a boot worthy of respect as confidence levels rise alongside with sense of empowerment, one repetition at a time!

WALL CALF RAISES FOR CALF DEFINITION AND STRENGTH

This specific exercise hones in on your calf muscles with precision, enabling you to attain a sculpted and toned appearance for your lower limbs. We will delve into the details of executing Wall Calf Raises professionally emphasizing their remarkable aesthetic benefits while offering invaluable tips for optimizing results.

Embarking on a routine that incorporates Wall Calf Raises serves as a game changer when it pertains to sculpting well defined calves; these exercises directly target the gastrocnemius and soleus muscles which compose a substantial segment of one's calves.

Leave behind shapeless calves and welcome confidently powerful contours for your lower limbs through incorporating this exercise into regular fitness sessions. Prepare yourself to unlock the full potential of these muscle groups so as to stride confidently in skirts, shorts or high heels that are dear to you!

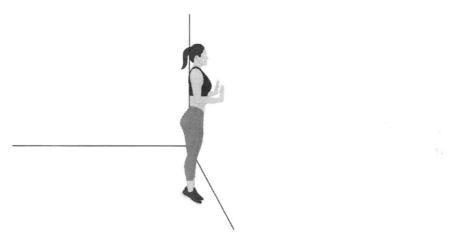

Step-by-Step Guide

1. Begin by standing facing a wall, approximately an arm's length away, with your feet hip-width apart and your hands resting against the wall for support.

2. Engage your core by drawing your navel towards your spine, and maintain a tall and proud posture throughout the exercise.

3. Slowly raise your heels off the ground, lifting your body onto the balls of your feet. Focus on contracting your calf muscles as you ascend.

4. Pause briefly at the top of the movement, feeling the stretch and contraction in your calves.

5. Lower your heels back down to the starting position in a controlled manner, allowing your calves to lengthen and stretch.

Tips

- Pay attention to proper form and alignment during wall calf raises. Keep your feet parallel and avoid letting your ankles roll inward or outward.

- Engage your calf muscles throughout the exercise, focusing on a strong and controlled contraction as you lift your heels.

- Breathe naturally throughout the movement, exhaling as you lift your heels and inhaling as you lower them.

- Keep your movements smooth and controlled, avoiding any sudden jerking or bouncing.

- Gradually increase the number of repetitions or sets as your calf strength improves.

Progression

Once you have mastered the basic Wall Calf Raises, you can challenge yourself by incorporating variations and progressions to further enhance your calf strength and definition. Here are a few options:

- **Single-Leg Wall Calf Raises:** Perform the calf raises on one leg at a time, focusing on maintaining balance and stability. This variation targets each calf individually and increases the intensity of the exercise.

- **Calf Raises with Added Weight:** Hold a dumbbell or a weighted object in one hand or use a calf raise machine to increase the resistance and challenge your calf muscles further.

- **Calf Raises on an Elevated Surface:** Place the balls of your feet on a step or an elevated platform, allowing your heels to lower below the level of your toes. This variation increases the range of motion and intensifies the calf muscle engagement. It's scientifically proven that working a muscle emphasizing the maximum stretch position of its range of motion, led to the best stimulus and results.

Incorporating Wall Calf Raises consistently into your fitness routine can bring about remarkable aesthetic benefits. Your calves will witness enhanced definition, toning, and shaping resulting in a sculpted athletic appearance for your lower legs. Imagine confidently displaying well-defined calves be it when wearing heels or showcasing them through athletic attire choices.

Embrace the burn that accompanies this exercise as well as embrace the challenges faced along the way; allow both to motivate you, serving as a catalyst for reaching new personal records.

Being a personal trainer who respects your determination, I have immense faith in your resiliency, ability to focus on objectives set while acknowledging difficulties, along with an unshakable belief in achieving remarkable outcomes through consistent efforts taken. Let this journey sculpt your lower legs into one's worthy of admiration, commanding attention from others while bestowing upon yourself unwavering confidence simultaneously.

Prepare yourself mentally and physically for surpassing previous limits reached; brace yourself for reaching new heights when it comes to redefining calf aesthetics!

WALL LEG SWINGS FOR HIP MOBILITY AND STABILITY

Are you interested in improving both your hip mobility and overall stability? If so, then look no further than the wonderful exercise known as Wall Leg Swings.

This particular exercise is designed to specifically target your hip muscles in order to enhance flexibility, range of motion, as well as stability. Wall Leg Swings are highly recommended for those wishing to boost their hip mobility as well as stability levels noticeably over time. By incorporating controlled leg swings, you can effectively engage the muscles surrounding the hips, including not only the hip flexors but also other major muscle groups essential for proper function, such as the abductors and adductors.

The movements performed throughout this exercise will not only help improve your range of motion but also contribute significantly towards attaining a more solid foundation for your lower body. Such improvements ultimately leading toward improved abilities both functional as well aesthetic.

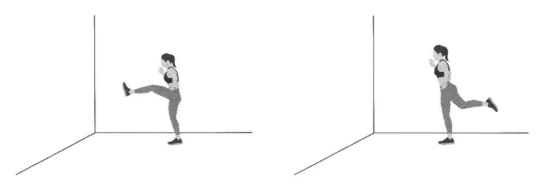

Step-by-Step Guide

1. Position yourself standing with your right side next to the wall (approximately an arm's length away), with your feet hip-width apart and your right hand resting against the wall for support.

2. Engage your core by drawing your navel towards your spine, and maintain a tall and proud posture throughout the exercise.

3. Begin by swinging your right leg forward and backward, allowing it to freely move within a comfortable range of motion.

4. Control the swing by using your hip muscles to initiate and control the movement. Focus on keeping the swinging motion smooth and controlled.

5. After completing the desired number of repetitions, switch side to swinging your left leg forward and backward, following the same controlled movement pattern.

Tips

- Maintain proper form and alignment during wall leg swings. Keep your standing leg slightly bent to support your body and provide stability.

- Engage your core muscles to help maintain balance and control throughout the exercise.

- Focus on a controlled and fluid movement, avoiding any jerking or swinging momentum that may compromise your form.

- Breathe naturally throughout the exercise, exhaling as you swing your leg forward and inhaling as you swing it backward.

- Keep your swinging leg relaxed and mobile, allowing the movement to come from your hip joint.

- Start with smaller swings and gradually increase the range of motion as your hip mobility improves.

- If you feel any discomfort or strain in your hip or lower back, decrease the range of motion or consult with a healthcare professional before continuing.

Progression

Once you have mastered the basic Wall Leg Swings, you can challenge yourself by incorporating variations and progressions to further enhance your hip mobility and stability. Here are a few options to consider:

- **Lateral Wall Leg Swings:** Instead of swinging your leg forward and backward, swing it out to the side and back, targeting your hip abductors. This variation improves your hip stability and adds a dynamic challenge to your workout. In this variation, position yourself with your back facing the wall.

- **Diagonal Wall Leg Swings:** Swing your leg in a diagonal motion, crossing it in front of your body and back out to the side. This variation targets different muscle groups around the hips and enhances your overall hip mobility and stability.

- **Single-Leg Wall Leg Swings:** Perform the swings while standing on one leg, without the support of the wall, focusing on maintaining your balance and stability throughout the movement. This variation enhances your stability and strengthens the supporting leg.

One can witness incredible aesthetic benefits by consistently incorporating Wall Leg Swings into their fitness routine. As a result, increased mobility in their hips allows for greater ease and grace during movements. For instance, envisioning oneself confidently striding forward while feeling both freedom and strength in their hips can truly enhance the transformative effects of this exercise. Inviting challenges while embracing fluidity is key to achieving new levels of hip mobility and stability.

Nevertheless, every swing presents an opportunity to connect with and strengthen your hip muscles. So, embrace the flow as well as the journey ahead for letting such transformative power empower you throughout new accomplishments.

5. UPPER BODY AND BACK EXERCISES

Greetings! Step into the splendid realm where you will discover a plethora of captivating pursuits that invigorate both your mind & muscles - welcome to the world of exquisite upper body & back exercises!

As we embark on this scintillating expedition together; redirect your focus towards sculpting & strengthening vital areas such as chest, arms and back region; unleashing dynamism with support from a simple wall.

Experience the benefits of targeted exercises designed to strengthen muscle groups and improve overall stability. Dive deeper into a variety of engaging wall exercises, including invigorating Wall Push-Ups, Triceps Push-Ups awe inspiring Wall and the energizing Wall Reverse Fly. Reinvent the essence of a vivacious upper physique simply engaging these prodigious moves, rendering you invincible! Bear in mind that attaining progress requires endurance over time alongside steadfastness in consistency.

Treat each exercise as an occasion for self-challenge which propels personal growth towards becoming an improved version of oneself. Allow yourself to wholeheartedly welcome both exertion at stake as well as accompanying hardships comprising this journey; knowing well their profound ability to inspire magnificent elevations within oneself.

In forthcoming sections, we are going to undertake an in-depth examination of each exercise, offering detailed guidelines, insightful suggestions, and adaptable modifications ensuring precise posture and execution.

May we now embark upon this captivating expedition together, one devoted to crafting and invigorating your chest, arms, upper back, and shoulders with utmost grace and finesse. Prepare yourself for the invigorating empowerment and unyielding confidence bestowed by a breath-taking sculpted upper body.

WALL PUSH-UPS FOR CHEST, ARM, AND CORE STRENGTH

Are you prepared to sculpt and enhance your chest, arms, and core? The wall Push-Ups are the perfect exercise for you. This workout makes use of a walls' support to target and engage multiple muscle groups effectively providing exceptional aesthetic advantages along with functional strength gains.

Wall Push-Ups represent an incredible exercise that aids in developing upper body strength specifically focusing on the chest, arms, as well as core areas. By making use of a walls support system combined with proper technique during each repetition session will prompt gradual increments in workout intensity while advancing over time to experience enhanced muscular gains and tonification. Get ready to unleash your upper body's power & grace through these exercises while observing their transformative impact on your physique.

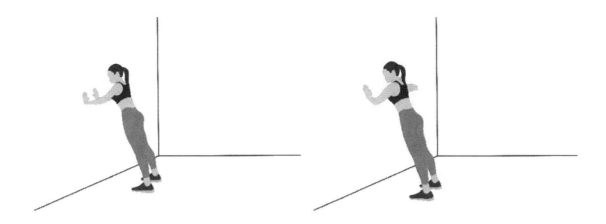

Step-by-Step Guide

1. Stand facing a wall with your feet hip-width apart, approximately an arm's length away from the wall.

2. Place your palms flat against the wall at chest height, slightly wider than shoulder-width apart. Your arms should be fully extended, and your body should be in a straight line from head to heels.

3. Engage your core muscles by drawing your navel towards your spine, and maintain a tall and proud posture throughout the exercise.

4. Bend your elbows and lower your chest towards the wall, keeping your body in a straight line. Focus on maintaining a controlled and slow descent.

5. Once your chest reaches the wall, push through your palms and extend your arms, returning to the starting position. Maintain a strong and stable core throughout the movement.

6. Repeat the movement for the desired number of repetitions, focusing on maintaining proper form and engaging the targeted muscles throughout the exercise.

Tips

- Maintain proper form and alignment during wall push-ups. Keep your body in a straight line from head to heels, and avoid arching or sagging your lower back.

- Engage your core muscles throughout the exercise to maintain stability and control.

- Focus on a controlled and slow descent, allowing your chest to approach the wall in a controlled manner.

- Exhale as you push away from the wall and inhale as you lower your chest towards the wall.

- Keep your elbows slightly tucked in towards your sides, avoiding flaring them out to the sides.

- Gradually increase the number of repetitions or sets as your upper body strength improves.

Progression

After acquiring enough skill in the fundamental Wall Push-Ups, you can opt to expand your repertoire by incorporating diverse variations and progressions. By delving into these advanced techniques, one can cultivate superior upper body strength while simultaneously enhancing muscle definition. Below are several viable options worth exploring:

- **Incline Wall Push-Ups:** Perform the push-ups with your hands placed higher on the wall, allowing for a greater challenge and increased engagement of your chest and arms.

- **Decline Wall Push-Ups:** Elevate your feet on a stable platform, such as a step or a bench, while performing the push-ups against the wall. This variation shifts more weight onto your upper body, intensifying the exercise.

- **Single-Leg Wall Push-Ups:** Lift one foot off the ground and perform the push-ups with one leg extended behind you. This variation challenges your core stability and increases the demand on your upper body muscles.

Through consistent integration of Wall Push-Ups into your current fitness regimen, expect nothing short of remarkable aesthetic benefits! Both your chest area and arm muscles will witness significant strength gains leading you towards achieving a toned and finely sculpted upper body.

Envision yourself exuding confidence while showcasing those well-defined chest and arms; feel free to flaunt them either in a stylish sleeveless top or perhaps even throughout summer months by the pool or beachside.

Always prioritize body awareness: listen attentively to its signals, respecting established boundaries on intensity levels while gradually scaling up exercise challenges further during each progressive milestone achieved. Always remember that each repetition is an opportunity that motivates personal growth, pushing both physical and emotional boundaries, leading to a truly transformative experience.

WALL TRICEPS PUSH-UPS FOR ARM DEFINITION AND TONE

Welcome to an effective arm toning exercise: Wall Triceps Push-Ups! This specific exercise hones in on your triceps muscles to help you achieve impressive arm definition and tone. By utilizing a supportive wall during this exercise, you can maintain proper form for maximal effectiveness.

This section provides a detailed guide on executing perfect Wall Triceps Push-Ups while emphasizing their exceptional benefits and offering valuable tips for optimal results. Prepare yourself for an extraordinary transformation in sculpting and toning your arms through this exercise! Your upper arms backside is home to the essential triceps muscles which significantly contribute to your overall arm strength and definition. Including regular sets of Wall Triceps Push-Ups in your workout routine efficiently targets these crucial muscles leading you towards beautifully toned arms that radiate confidence.

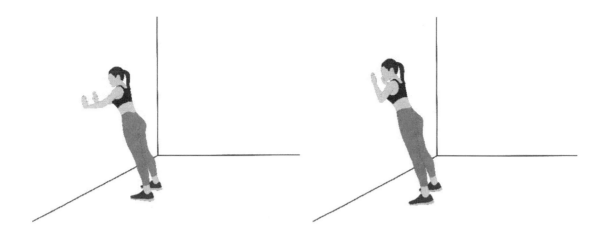

Step-by-Step Guide

1. Stand facing a wall with your feet hip-width apart, approximately an arm's length away from the wall.

2. Place your palms flat against the wall, slightly lower than shoulder height and shoulder-width apart. Your arms should be fully extended, and your body should form a straight line from head to heels.

3. Engage your core by drawing your navel towards your spine and maintaining a tall and proud posture throughout the exercise.

4. Bend your elbows and lean towards the wall, keeping your body in a straight line. Focus on maintaining a controlled and slow descent.

5. Once your elbows reach a 90-degree angle, push through your palms and extend your arms, returning to the starting position. Keep your core strong and stable throughout the movement.

6. Repeat the movement for the desired number of repetitions, focusing on maintaining proper form and engaging your triceps throughout the exercise.

Tips

- Maintain proper form and alignment during wall triceps push-ups. Keep your body in a straight line from head to heels and avoid arching or sagging your lower back.

- Engage your core muscles throughout the exercise to maintain stability and control.

- Focus on a controlled and slow descent, allowing your elbows to bend to a 90-degree angle.

- Exhale as you push away from the wall and inhale as you lower your body towards the wall.

- Keep your elbows close to your sides, avoiding flaring them outwards.

- Gradually increase the number of repetitions or sets as your triceps strength improves.

Progression

As you build strength and become more comfortable with Wall Triceps Push-Ups, you can increase the challenge by incorporating the following progressions:

- **Diamond Wall Push-Ups:** Place your hands close together on the wall, forming a diamond shape with your fingers. This variation emphasizes triceps engagement to a greater extent.

- **Triceps Dips on a Chair:** Find a stable chair or elevated surface and position your hands on the edge with your fingers pointing towards your body. Lower your body towards the ground by bending your elbows and then push back up. This variation adds more resistance to your triceps.

For remarkable aesthetic benefits consider incorporating Wall Triceps Push-Ups into your regular fitness routine. This will result in more defined, toned and sculpted arms that will boost your confidence when proudly wearing sleeveless tops or dresses.

Take a moment to envision yourself confidently showing off your beautifully sculpted arms wherever life takes you. Each triceps push-up brings an opportunity for personal growth allowing for increased strength while transforming those arm muscles – so embrace that burn! Let these incredible Wall Triceps Push-Ups inspire you towards reaching new heights by accepting their challenge wholeheartedly.

Together, with your dedication, consistency, and the right mindset, we can unlock the full potential of your triceps and create the arms you've always dreamt of. Embrace this exciting adventure to tone your triceps and experience the feelings of strength, confidence, and empowerment that lie ahead.

WALL ROWS FOR BACK SCULPTING

Would you like to strengthen and tone your upper back while also improving your posture? If so, Wall Rows is the perfect exercise for you. This particular exercise focuses on the muscles in your upper back helping you achieve a pleasing and confident posture. By incorporating Wall Rows into your workout routine, you can strengthen and shape your upper back while enjoying the many benefits of improved posture.

Wall Rows are truly transformative when it comes to developing a strong and well-defined upper back. As already mentioned, the muscles in this area play a crucial role in maintaining proper posture, but also shoulder stability and overall strength in the upper body. In fact, through the practice of Wall Rows, you can effectively target and engage these muscles, leading to improved posture and a more sculpted upper back. Prepare yourself to unleash the potential within your upper back and experience the confidence that accompanies better and upright posture.

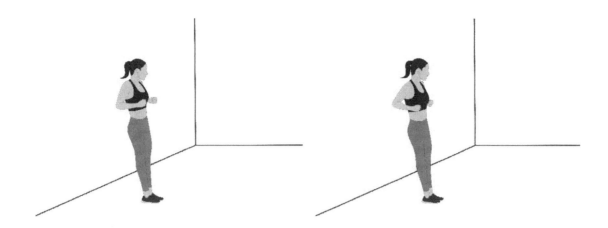

Step-by-Step Guide

1. Begin by standing with your back against the wall with your feet shoulder-width apart, approximately an arm's length away from the wall, and your knees slightly bent.

2. Raise your elbows until they are about 45 degrees apart from your torso, keeping them flat against the wall while your forearms are perpendicular to the wall.

3. Engage your core muscles by drawing your navel toward your spine, and maintain a tall and proud posture throughout the exercise.

4. Keeping your body in a straight line from head to heels, slowly push your elbows against the wall and pull your body away from the wall. Imagine squeezing your shoulder blades together as you perform the movement.

5. Pause for a moment when your upper back is at the maximum distance from the wall, then slowly return to the starting position, maintaining control and engaging your upper back muscles throughout.

6. Repeat the movement for the desired number of repetitions, focusing on maintaining proper form and feeling the engagement in your upper back muscles.

Tips

- Focus on maintaining proper form and alignment throughout the exercise. Keep your body in a straight line, avoiding any arching or sagging of the lower back.

- Imagine pulling your elbows back and squeezing your shoulder blades together as you perform the rowing motion. This will ensure that you are targeting the correct muscles and maximizing the effectiveness of the exercise.

- Keep your shoulders relaxed and away from your ears throughout the movement. Avoid shrugging or tensing your upper body.

- Control the movement both on the way up and on the way down, emphasizing the engagement of your upper back muscles throughout the entire range of motion.

- Breathe naturally throughout the exercise, exhaling as you pull your body toward the wall and inhaling as you extend your arms.

- Gradually increase the number of repetitions or sets as your upper back strength improves.

Progression

If the basic Wall Rows start to be too easy, you may wish to push yourself by incorporating different variations and progressions. This will aid in improving your upper back strength and definition. Below are several options for you:

- **Single-Arm Wall Rows:** Perform the rows with one arm at a time, alternating between arms. This variation increases the demand on each side of the upper back and improves muscular balance.

- **Resistance Band Wall Rows:** Instead of lying your back on the wall, attach a resistance band to the wall or a sturdy anchor point (roughly at the height of your shoulders), position yourself in front of the wall and perform the rows while holding onto the band handles. This provides additional resistance, challenging your upper back and lats muscles further. In this case, your starting position will be with your arms extended in front of you, parallel to the floor. As you pull the band focus on a "rowing" movement: think of how you should bring you elbows down to your hips. The movement ends when your arms are aligned with your body.

- **Weighted Wall Rows:** Hold a dumbbell or kettlebell in each hand while performing the rows: maintaining a straight back, lean forward until your body is inclined about 45 degrees. Perform the rows as described in the Resistance Band Wall Rows variation, focusing on bringing your elbows down to your hips. This adds an extra challenge and promotes greater muscle activation. You can perform this exercise with one hand at a time, placing the palm of the free hand flat against the wall to ensure a proper balance.

By incorporating Wall Rows consistently into your fitness routine, you will witness extraordinary aesthetic benefits. Strengthening your whole back will result in it being more defined and sculpted while also enhancing your posture for a more confident presence.

Picture yourself standing tall with proud composure radiating strength combined with gracefulness. Remember to listen attentively to your body's signals while respecting its limitations; gradually increase intensity levels over time as well as exercise difficulty as warranted by progress made. Aspire for reaching new heights through embracing both sweat-inducing burnings sensation along with encountering difficult challenges associated with performing these exercises! Be prepared for such dedication reflecting itself when exhibiting confidence by carrying yourself in a poised manner while enjoying all incredible advantages that are offered by engaging regularly in practicing this unique exercise.

WALL SHOULDER PRESS

Welcome to the captivating world of Wall Shoulder Press! This empowering exercise has been designed specifically with the aim of targeting your shoulder muscles, thereby assisting you in building strength, stability and defining this crucial area.

By incorporating Wall Shoulder Presses into your regular training routine, not only will you be able to achieve astounding aesthetic benefits, but you will also enhance your overall upper body strength and functionality simultaneously. Wall Shoulder Presses essentially emerge as an extraordinary exercise when it comes to developing powerful looking sculpted shoulders that project an air of confidence.

It is important to recognize that the muscles in our shoulders like deltoids along with all interconnected stabilizers play a pivotal role in executing diverse movements associated with our upper bodies as a whole. Thus, firmly contributing toward enhancing aesthetics across our upper halves too! Simply by incorporating Wall Shoulder Presses into our workout regimen consistently enough one can effectively have visible improvements, such as boosted strength levels along with finely toned definition across shoulders.

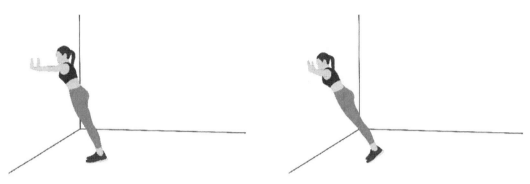

Step-by-Step Guide

1. Stand facing a wall with your feet shoulder-width apart, approximately a step's length away from the wall.

2. Position your hands on the wall slightly wider than shoulder-width apart, at approximately shoulder height. Your palms should face forward, and your elbows should be slightly bent.

3. Engage your core muscles by drawing your navel toward your spine, and maintain a tall and proud posture throughout the exercise.

4. Inhale as you bend your elbows and lower your body toward the wall until your nose almost touches it, maintaining control and a slow, controlled tempo.

5. Exhale as you push your body away from the wall, extending your arms fully without locking your elbows. Focus on pressing through your shoulders and feeling the engagement in your shoulder muscles.

6. Repeat the movement for the desired number of repetitions, focusing on maintaining proper form and feeling the targeted muscles working.

Tips

- Maintain a slight bend in your elbows throughout the exercise to keep tension on the muscles and avoid excessive strain on the joints.

- Focus on quality over quantity. Perform the shoulder presses with control, emphasizing the contraction and extension of your shoulder muscles.

- Keep your shoulders relaxed and away from your ears throughout the movement. Avoid shrugging or tensing your upper body.

- Engage your core muscles to stabilize your body throughout the exercise. This will not only enhance your shoulder strength but also improve overall stability and balance.

- Breathe naturally throughout the exercise, exhaling as you push away from the wall and inhaling as you return to the starting position.

- Gradually increase the resistance or weight as your shoulder strength improves.

Progression

Once you have mastered the basic Wall Shoulder Press, you can test your abilities by introducing different variations and progressions that will elevate your shoulder strength and enhance their definition. Here are a few alternatives for you to contemplate upon:

- **Single-Arm Wall Shoulder Press:** Perform the shoulder presses with one arm at a time, alternating between arms. Keep the not-working arm behind your back or against the wall if you need more balance (note, if you keep your free hand on the wall, its only purpose is to ensure balance so don't push actively with it). This variation increases the demand on each shoulder individually and improves muscular balance.

- **Stability Ball Wall Shoulder Press:** Perform the shoulder presses while seated on a stability ball, engaging your core for added stability and engaging more muscle fibers throughout your body.

Incorporating Wall Shoulder Presses into your fitness routine consistently can lead to impressive improvements in appearance. Your shoulders will become stronger more defined, and sculpted, enhancing the overall look of your upper body.

Imagine the confidence you'll feel when you confidently wear sleeveless tops and proudly show off your well-defined shoulders. Get ready to embrace greatness by shouldering the weight with confidence that will speak for itself.

WALL REVERSE FLY FOR UPPER BACK SCULPTING

Step into the world of Wall Reverse Flies with open arms as I present you with an exceptional exercise that holds remarkable potential in sculpting and toning your upper back. This Pilates exercise serves as a valuable tool in achieving a firm, defined, and visually pleasing appearance that exudes confidence. By incorporating Wall Reverse Flies into your current regime, you can effectively target the major muscle groups found in your upper back, including the rhomboids, posterior deltoids and trapezius, creating a well-rounded physique that captivates others.

It is pertinent to note that by engaging in this fantastic exercise, growth can be witnessed not only aesthetically but also posturally. Indeed, sculpting one's muscular framework contributes not only towards cultivating symmetry within one's body but also boosts overall posture aligning it with strength and functionality whilst enhancing personal confidence levels significantly. Prepare yourself for this journey as we unlock the hidden splendor of your upper back through performing Wall Reverse Flies with proper form.

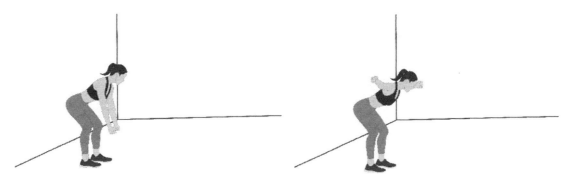

Step-by-Step Guide

1. Stand with your back facing a wall with your feet shoulder-width apart, approximately an arm's length away from the wall.

2. Lean your buttock against the wall and bend your torso forward keeping your spine neutral (don't arch it).

3. Your knees should be bent and keep your arms perpendicular to the floor, behind your legs. This is the starting position.

4. Engage your core muscles by drawing your navel toward your spine and maintain a tall and proud posture throughout the exercise.

5. Keeping your arms straight, exhale as you raise them squeezing your shoulder blades together and pull your hands away from the floor, moving them laterally toward the sides of your body until they are parallel to the floor.

6. Inhale as you slowly return your hands to the starting position, maintaining control and a slow, controlled tempo.

7. Repeat the movement for the desired number of repetitions, focusing on maintaining proper form and feeling the upper back and rear deltoids working.

Tips

*   Focus on the mind-muscle connection. Visualize and feel your upper back muscles working during each repetition to optimize their activation and engagement.

*   Keep your neck relaxed and in a neutral position throughout the exercise. Avoid straining or tensing your neck muscles.

- Control the movement and avoid using momentum. Perform the wall reverse flies in a slow and controlled manner, emphasizing the contraction and extension of your upper back muscles.

- Imagine squeezing a pencil between your shoulder blades as you pull your hands away from the floor. This mental cue can help you engage the targeted muscles more effectively.

- Maintain proper posture and alignment throughout the exercise. Avoid rounding your shoulders or slouching forward. Imagine a string pulling you upward from the crown of your head.

- Breathe naturally throughout the exercise, exhaling as you squeeze your shoulder blades together and inhaling as you return to the starting position.

- Gradually increase the difficulty of the exercise by incorporating resistance bands or using lighter weights. A simple trick to add weight to this exercise is to hold a little bottle of water in each hand.

Progression

After mastering the basic Wall Reverse Flies, you can further enhance your upper back strength and definition by incorporating variations and progressions. Here are some options to consider:

- **Resistance Band Wall Reverse Flies:** Hold a resistance band in your hands, in this variation, position straight-tall with your back against the wall. Start with your arms straight in front of you, parallel to the floor with the palms of your hands facing down. Perform the reverse flies while maintaining tension on the band throughout the movement as you move your hands away until your arms are aligned with your body, thus touching the wall. This increases resistance and intensifies the exercise.

- **Unilateral Wall Reverse Flies:** Perform the reverse flies with one arm at a time, focusing on engaging and strengthening each side of your upper back individually. This helps improve muscular balance and symmetry. Remember, if you want to add more difficulty, hold a little weight in your hands like small water bottles.

- **Wall Reverse Fly with External Rotation:** Perform the reverse fly movement, but as you pull your hands up, rotate your arms externally, so your palms face upward. This engages additional muscles and adds a rotational component to the exercise.

If you consistently integrate Wall Reverse Flies into your upper body training routine, an exquisitely sculpted and well-defined upper back that complements your overall physique can be yours to behold. Consider the confidence boost and sense of accomplishment that will wash over you as soon as your back becomes notably stronger, beautifully toned, and undeniably captivating. Get ready to fully embrace this challenge; with dedication comes progress beyond measure.

Your remarkable transformation lies just ahead - are you prepared? Sink into consistent practice sessions, maintain a positive mindset throughout thus enabling yourself to fully unleash the immense potential hidden within your upper back muscles. Prepare to witness astounding aesthetic results that will leave you breathless. As a personal trainer committed to supporting people like you, I wish you to spread your wings wide and soar towards newfound levels of strength, beauty, and self-confidence.

6. TOTAL BODY EXERCISES

I wholeheartedly welcome you to embark on an exhilarating journey within the enchanting realm of total body exercises!

Throughout this chapter lies an assortment of dynamic and stimulating movements that concurrently engage multiple muscle groups simultaneously. These meticulously curated exercises have been crafted to administer an exhaustive workout targeting your entire body. With the incorporation of these exercises into your regimen, you can anticipate a comprehensive enhancement in your overall strength, cardiovascular endurance, stability, as well as fat burning. Prepare yourself to luxuriate in a fitness approach that combines mind, body and soul by acquainting yourself with wall-based total body exercises.

When it comes to achieving a harmonious and functional physique, total body integration exercises epitomize the pinnacle of efficiency and efficacy. By initiating synchronized movements involving various muscle groups these exercises optimize training time while delivering extraordinary results. Every exercise highlighted within this chapter has been strategically chosen to specifically target crucial areas of your body, including (but not limited to) the core, shoulders, hamstrings, obliques as well as hips. By incorporating them into your routine you will unwrap a transformative workout experience that challenges your physicality in fresh and intriguing ways.

Whether you aspire for burgeoning strength or amplified cardiovascular endurance, whether improved stability or bolstered power is what fuels your passion, rest assured! The total body integration exercises presented within this chapter encompass all of these aspirations and beyond. They are designed with utmost care so that they address every aspect of your holistic fitness journey taking you above and beyond, granting you the balanced physique enriched with functionality that you deeply crave.

Continuing on our voyage through the mesmerizing world of total body exercises, let's provide an overview of each featured exercise, highlighting their individual benefits alongside the challenges they bestow upon. These hand-picked exercises are crafted to stretch limits, set aflame dormant muscles while revitalizing ones' very spirit. Without further ado, let us venture together into this astounding universe where total body activation reigns supreme.

WALL PIKE FOR CORE, SHOULDER, AND HAMSTRING STRENGTH

I extend a warm welcome as you enter into the captivating world of Wall Pike! This particular exercise serves as an exceptional tool for developing strength in vital areas such as your core muscles, shoulders, and hamstrings.

By seamlessly integrating Wall Pike into your regular workout regimen, a wealth of marvellous benefits lie within reach that can facilitate attaining an aesthetic physique characterized by toned muscles and overall balance.

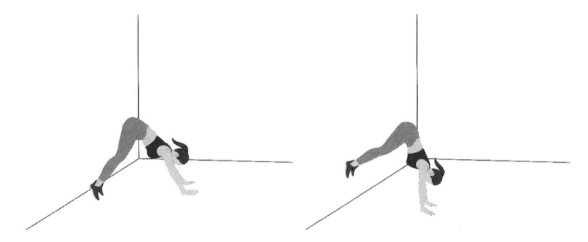

Step-by-Step Guide

1. Begin by standing with your back facing the wall, approximately an arm's length away. Place your hands on the floor in front of you, shoulder-width apart, and walk your feet up the wall until your body forms an inverted "V" shape. Note, if this position is too challenging for you, you can lay your whole forearm to the floor instead of only your palms.

2. Engage your core muscles by drawing your navel toward your spine. Keep your arms straight and your shoulders strong and stable throughout the exercise.

3. Inhale deeply, then exhale as you lift your hips towards the ceiling, pressing your feet into the wall. Your body should form a straight line from your hands to your hips.

4. Pause at the top for a moment, feeling the engagement in your core, shoulders, and hamstrings. Keep this position for 5 seconds squeezing your core.

5. Inhale as you slowly lower your hips back down to the starting position, maintaining control and stability throughout the movement.

6. Repeat for the desired number of repetitions, focusing on maintaining proper form and feeling the targeted muscles working.

Tips

- Maintain a strong plank position throughout the exercise, keeping your core engaged and your back straight.

- Focus on pressing your feet into the wall to activate your hamstrings and maximize the benefits for your lower body.

- Keep your shoulders away from your ears and avoid shrugging. Focus on keeping them stable and engaged throughout the movement.

- Breathe deeply and rhythmically throughout the exercise, inhaling as you lower your hips and exhaling as you lift them.

Progression

Once you have mastered the basic Wall Pike, you can challenge yourself further by incorporating these progressions:

- **Pike Push-Ups:** Perform a push-up while in the Wall Pike position. This variation adds an extra challenge for your upper body strength and shoulder stability.

- **Single-Leg Wall Pike:** Lift one leg off the wall (trying to raise it perpendicular to the ground) while performing the Wall Pike, alternating between legs. This variation increases the demand on your core stability enhancing balance and adding a glute squeezing component.

The Wall Pike exercise is a movement that targets key areas of your body including your core, shoulders and hamstrings. It provides a workout that not enhances strength but also improves aesthetics. By following the step by step guide, implementing tips and gradually progressing, you can fully unlock the potential of this exercise. Achieve amazing results: get ready to feel empowered, strong and confident as you strengthen your core sculpt your shoulders and enhance the flexibility and strength of your hamstrings. Embracing this challenge maintaining consistency and enjoying the journey will help transform your body and achieve your fitness goals.

WALL MOUNTAIN CLIMBERS FOR CARDIOVASCULAR ENDURANCE AND CORE ACTIVATION

Let's step into the realm of Wall Mountain Climbers! This exercise offers a thrilling and demanding motion that not enhances your endurance but also engages and reinforces your core muscles. By integrating Wall Mountain Climbers into your exercise regimen, you can unlock an array of advantages such, as heightened stamina, fortified core stability and a sculpted midsection.

In this segment I will furnish you with an expert guide on executing Wall Mountain Climbers complete, with instructions, indispensable pointers and advanced techniques to propel your fitness expedition to unparalleled levels. Are you ready to feel the burn?

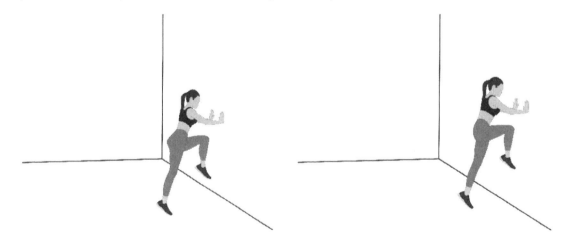

Step-by-Step Guide

1. Start by facing the wall in a push-up position with your hands flat against the wall, slightly wider than shoulder-width apart.

2. Engage your core muscles by drawing your navel toward your spine. Maintain a strong and stable plank position throughout the exercise.

3. Begin by driving one knee toward your chest, lifting your foot off the ground and towards the wall.

4. Quickly switch legs, bringing the lifted leg back to the starting position while driving the opposite knee towards your chest.

5. Continue alternating legs in a rhythmic and controlled manner, maintaining a steady pace.

6. Focus on keeping your hips level and avoiding any excessive twisting or swaying of the body.

7. Aim for a smooth and fluid motion, as if you are running against the wall.

Tips

- Keep your core muscles engaged throughout the exercise. Imagine drawing your belly button towards your spine to maintain stability and control.

- Maintain a strong and stable upper body position, avoiding any rounding or sagging of the shoulders. Keep your wrists aligned with your shoulders.

- Focus on your breath, inhaling deeply as you draw your knee towards your chest and exhaling as you extend your leg back.

- Keep your gaze focused on the wall to maintain proper alignment and avoid straining your neck.

Progression

Once you have mastered the basic Wall Mountain Climbers, you can challenge yourself further by incorporating these progressions:

- **Speed Variation:** Increase the tempo of your leg movements, performing the mountain climbers at a faster pace to elevate your heart rate and intensify the cardiovascular component of the exercise.

- **Knee-to-Elbow Mountain Climbers:** Instead of driving your knee towards your chest, aim to bring it towards the opposite elbow. This variation adds an extra challenge to your core muscles and further engages your obliques.

Wall Mountain Climbers offer a thrilling workout blending the benefits of endurance, core activation and fat burning potential. Adding this exercise to your fitness regimen allows you to attain a toned and sculpted midsection. Embrace the challenge it presents focus on executing the form and technique and relish the invigorating sensation of pushing yourself to new limits.

With unwavering consistency, effort and a positive mindset you can elevate your fitness levels enhance your endurance and witness transformations in your core aesthetics.

WALL SIDE PLANK WITH LEG LIFTS FOR OBLIQUE AND HIP STABILITY

Welcome to the world of Wall Side Plank with Leg Lifts! This exercise offers an avenue to focus on and fortify your muscles while simultaneously enhancing your hip stability. By integrating Wall Side Plank with Leg Lifts into your workout regimen, you can unlock a myriad of advantages such as defined and chiselled obliques, amplified core stability, refined balance and an intense glutes stimulus. In this segment, I will furnish you with an in depth and polished guide on executing Wall Side Plank with Leg Lifts. Well my dear, let's break down each step, providing indispensable pointers and progressions that will propel your fitness journey to new heights.

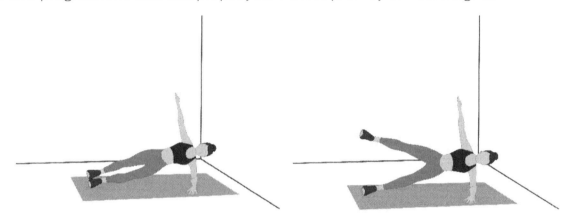

Step-by-Step Guide

1. Start by standing next to a wall with your head facing the wall. Place your forearm on the ground, perpendicular to your body, and position your elbow directly under your shoulder.

2. Extend your legs out to the side and position your feet against the wall. Your body should be in a straight line from your head to your feet.

3. Engage your core muscles by drawing your navel toward your spine. This will help stabilize your body throughout the exercise.

4. Lift your hips off the ground, creating a straight line from your shoulders to your ankles. This is the starting position for the Wall Side Plank.

5. Once you have established a stable side plank position, lift your top leg off the floor, maintaining control and balance. Take advantage of the proximity to the wall to maintain a straight trajectory as you lift your leg, avoiding moving it from the line of your body.

6. Slowly lower your leg back down to the floor, keeping your hips lifted and your body aligned.

7. Repeat the leg lift movement for the desired number of repetitions, maintaining proper form and engaging your oblique muscles.

Tips

- Focus on maintaining a strong and stable side plank position throughout the exercise. Avoid letting your hips drop or sag.

- Keep your core muscles engaged by imagining that you are pulling your waistline up towards the ceiling.

- Pay attention to your breathing. Inhale as you prepare for the leg lift, and exhale as you lift your leg and lower it back down.

- Keep your neck in a neutral position, aligning it with the rest of your spine. Avoid straining or tensing your neck muscles.

- Control the movement of your leg lifts and avoid using momentum. Focus on engaging your oblique muscles to lift and lower your leg.

Progression

Once you have mastered the basic Wall Side Plank with Leg Lifts, you can challenge yourself further by incorporating these progressions:

- **Extended Arm Variation:** Instead of placing your forearm on the ground, extend your arm fully and position your hand flat against the floor. This variation increases the stability challenge and further engages your shoulder muscles.

- **Knee-to-Elbow Side Plank:** From the side plank position, bring your top elbow and knee together, engaging your oblique muscles even more intensely. This variation adds a rotational component and targets your obliques from a different angle.

The Wall Side Plank with Leg Lifts is an effective way to target and strengthen your muscles while also promoting hip slimming and stability. When you incorporate this exercise into your fitness routine, you'll notice results like toned and sculpted obliques, enhanced core stability and awesome glutes tonification. Embracing the challenge of this exercise focusing on form and technique will ensure you enjoy the feeling of a strong and stable side plank.

Let the Wall Side Plank with Leg Lifts be your guide to a more balanced body and always remember, you possess the power to achieve results and unlock the best version of yourself!

WALL SPIDERMAN PLANK FOR TOTAL BODY ENGAGEMENT AND CORE STRENGTH

Engaging in this exercise offers a stimulating workout that involves your body focusing on strengthening your core and burning tons of calories. By including the Wall Spiderman Plank in your fitness regimen, you can reap advantages such as boosting core strength, refining balance augmenting both upper and lower body power and achieving a fit physique. Here I present an expertly crafted guide on executing the Wall Spiderman Plank. It will furnish you with step by step instructions, vital tips and progressive variations to elevate your fitness endeavors.

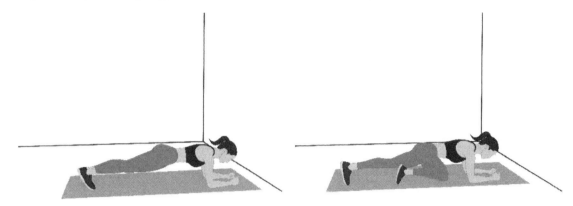

Step-by-Step Guide

1. Start by lying down to the floor and place your hands flat on the floor, slightly wider than shoulder-width apart.

2. Step your feet back and lift your body onto the balls of your feet, creating a plank position. Your body should form a straight line from your head to your heels.

3. Engage your core muscles by drawing your navel toward your spine. This will help stabilize your body throughout the exercise.

4. As you hold the plank position, bend your right knee and bring it toward your right elbow, aiming to touch or get as close as possible.

5. Return your right leg to the starting position and repeat the movement on the opposite side, bringing your left knee toward your left elbow.

6. Continue alternating the Spiderman knee drive, maintaining a strong and stable plank position.

Tips

- Focus on maintaining proper form and alignment throughout the exercise. Keep your body in a straight line, avoiding sagging or arching your lower back.

- Engage your core muscles throughout the movement. Imagine drawing your belly button toward your spine and creating tension in your abdominal muscles.

- Keep your shoulders down and away from your ears. Avoid shrugging or tensing your neck and shoulder muscles.

- Breathe steadily throughout the exercise. Inhale deeply as you prepare, and exhale as you drive your knee toward your elbow.

- Control the movement and avoid using momentum. Perform the Spiderman knee drive in a slow and controlled manner, emphasizing the engagement of your core and the stability of your plank position.

Progression

Once you have mastered the basic Wall Spiderman Plank, you can further enhance your workout routine by incorporating the following progressions:

- **Spiderman Push-ups:** Perform a push-up after each Spiderman knee drive. This adds an upper body strength element to the exercise and further engages your chest, shoulders, and triceps.

- **Wall Spiderman Plank with Leg Extension:** After bringing your knee toward your elbow, extend your leg straight out behind you, parallel to the ground. This variation increases the demand on your core muscles and adds an element of balance and stability.

The Wall Spiderman Plank is an exercise that engages entirely your body, strengthens your core and let you burning a significant number of calories. Adding this movement to your training routine can yield numerous benefits, including improved core stability, better balance, greater lower body strength and a sculpted, toned physique. Hug the challenge focus on maintaining form and technique and relish the empowering sensation of a stable plank.

Embrace the journey stay committed and let the incredible benefits of the Wall Spiderman Plank guide you towards becoming a fitter and more self-assured version of yourself. Keep pushing and embrace the strength within you!

WALL BURPEES FOR FULL-BODY CONDITIONING AND POWER

Let's step in the world of Wall Burpees! This compound movement is a demanding exercise that engages your entire body giving you a robust and comprehensive conditioning session. Adding Wall Burpees to your training routine brings forth advantages: boosting your fitness enhancing muscular strength and endurance also amplifying explosive power as well as sculpting and toning your physique by a demanding cardio activity.

Wall Burpees are one of the most complete exercises, a game changer if you aim aesthetic goals. They go beyond giving you a total body workout by targeting very eye-catching muscle groups particularly for women seeking a toned, sculpted, and visually appealing physique. So look at this exercise as a real asset in your journey, towards obtaining a confident and aesthetically pretty body.

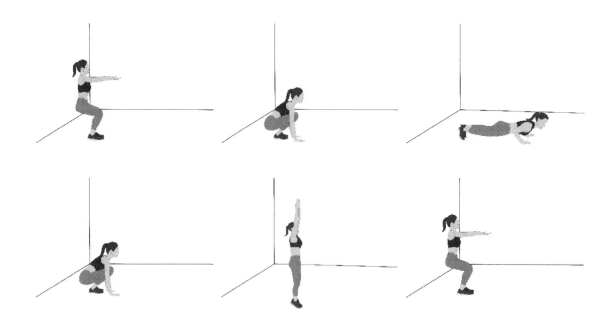

Step-by-Step Guide

1. Stand with your back facing a wall, approximately a step's length away. Place your feet shoulder-width apart, maintaining a strong and stable posture.

2. Begin the movement by lowering your body into a squat position, bending at the hips and knees. Keep your chest lifted and your weight in your heels.

3. Place your hands on the floor in front of you, shoulder-width apart, and slightly wider than your shoulders.

4. Kick your feet back, extending your legs behind you, and land in a push-up position with your body forming a straight line from head to heels.

5. Perform a push-up by bending your elbows and lowering your chest toward the floor. Keep your core engaged and your body stable throughout the movement.

6. Explosively jump your feet forward, landing in a squat position as close to the wall as possible. Use your legs and core to generate power and height in the jump.

7. From the squat position, jump vertically, reaching your arms overhead toward the ceiling.

8. Land softly, absorbing the impact through your legs, and immediately transition into the next repetition.

Tips

- Focus on maintaining proper form and alignment throughout the exercise. Keep your core engaged, your back straight, and your movements controlled.

- Engage your core muscles to stabilize your body during the squat, push-up, and jump phases of the exercise.

- Land softly and quietly to reduce the impact on your joints. Use your leg muscles to absorb the landing and maintain control.

- Breathe deeply and consistently throughout the exercise. Inhale during the descent and exhale during the explosive phases of the movement.

- Control the movement and avoid rushing through the exercise. Perform each repetition with intention and focus on quality over quantity.

- Start with a modified version if needed. Instead of kicking your feet back into a push-up position, step one foot back at a time and then step them back in during the jump phase.

- If the toe on the floor push-up position is too challenging for you, try laying on your knees instead.

- Gradually increase the intensity by incorporating variations and progressions, such as adding a clap overhead during the jump or performing the exercise with a weighted vest.

Progression

Once you have mastered the basic Wall Burpee, you can challenge yourself by incorporating these progressions:

- **Plyometric Wall Burpees:** Instead of a vertical jump, perform a tuck jump by bringing your knees toward your chest during the jump phase. This adds an explosive element and increases the intensity of the exercise.

- **Wall Burpee with Push-up:** After kicking your feet back into the push-up position, perform a full push-up before jumping your feet forward and into the squat position. This variation adds an extra challenge for your upper body and core muscles.

- **Plank Jack Burpees:** Perform a burpee as usual, but when you are in the push-up position, jump your feet wide and then back together, mimicking a jumping jack motion. This version targets your inner and outer thighs, adding more intensity to your workout and engaging additional muscle groups.

Wall Burpees and their variations provide a range of advantages that contribute to attaining a well-defined, sculpted and visually pleasing physique. By welcoming the challenge and integrating this exercise into your workout regimen you can witness improvements in endurance and a remarkable, stunning, transformation of your body.!

7. CREATING WORKOUT PLANS

Here we arrived to Chapter 7 of our journey. Here we delve into the realm of crafting workout plans that're not only effective but also captivating. This chapter aims to provide you with the know-how and resources for the creation of structured training programs that cater to your individual fitness level and aspirations. Whether you're a beginner looking to establish a foundation, an intermediate enthusiast eager to push your limits, or an advanced fitness enthusiast aiming to elevate your physical prowess, fear not!

This chapter encompasses it all; prepare yourself for an exhilarating and empowering workout encounter with my tailored Wall Pilates workout plans. It's time to take action!

FUNDAMENTALS FOR DESIGNING TRAINING PROGRAM

Before we dive into the workout plans it's crucial to grasp the basics of program design. In this section we'll explore the principles and important factors to consider when crafting a workout plan that truly delivers results. Whether your goal is to boost strength improve fitness or achieve an aesthetic goal, comprehending these foundational elements will set you on the path to success. So, let's embark on this journey! Uncover the secrets behind designing a training program that will propel you toward your dream shape.

Goal Setting

The first step in designing any training program is to clearly define your goals. Ask yourself, "What do I want to achieve?" Is it weight loss, muscle toning, increased strength, or improved overall fitness? Setting Specific, Measurable, Attainable, Relevant, and Time-bound (SMART) goals will provide direction and keep you focused throughout your fitness journey. In particular, the workout programs featured in this book have a dual focus: shedding excess weight and sculpting your physique. You see, achieving a stunning body isn't just about shedding those extra pounds; the real magic lies in "toning", which is achieved by a proper workout routine.

Assessing Your Current Fitness Level

To design a program that suits your abilities, it's crucial to assess your current fitness level. Evaluate your strength, endurance, flexibility, and any limitations or injuries you may have. This assessment will help you determine the starting point and progressions within your program. For this purpose, I suggest to start from the beginners' programs. If you'll find them too easy, jump in the intermediate ones, and so forth!

Determining Training Frequency

Consider how often you can commit to training each week. Consistency is key, so aim for a frequency that aligns with your schedule and allows for adequate recovery. For beginners, three to four sessions per week may be appropriate, while more experienced individuals may aim for four to six sessions.

Exercise Selection

Select exercises that align with your goals and target the specific muscle groups or energy systems you want to work on. Incorporate a mix of compound exercises (which engage multiple muscle groups) and isolation exercises (which target specific muscles). Focus on movements that are safe, effective, and enjoyable to keep you motivated. Well, for this aspect, you're in the right place!

Structuring Your Program

To optimize results, structure your program to include a variety of training modalities. This may include resistance training, cardiovascular exercises, flexibility work, and functional movements. Balance your workouts to address all major muscle groups and ensure overall body conditioning. Wall Pilates perfectly embodies all of these features.

Progressive Overload

To keep pushing your body and triggering those incredible changes, it's essential to embrace the principle of *progressive overload*. It entails a gradual increasing of the intensity, duration, or resistance of your workouts over time. This can be achieved by increasing repetitions or sets, shortening rest periods, or trying more challenging variations of exercises. But don't rush, let your body to properly adapt to the new stimuli before trying to increase them.

Rest and Recovery

Allowing your body adequate rest and recovery is just as important as the workout itself. Schedule rest days or active recovery sessions to prevent overtraining and support muscle repair and growth. Listen to your body and adjust your program if you experience excessive fatigue or signs of overuse.

Tracking Progress

Keep a record of your workouts to track your progress over time. This can be done through a training journal, mobile app, or spreadsheet. Monitoring your performance, strength gains, and changes in body composition will provide valuable feedback and help you make adjustments as needed.

Drawing from my extensive experience as a personal trainer, I'm thrilled to share some tips that can assist you in attaining the image you aspire for!

One crucial aspect is maintaining motivation by setting short term goals that contribute to your long-term objectives. It's essential to acknowledge and celebrate your accomplishments along the way as this foster continued enthusiasm and momentum.

Another vital strategy is embracing variety within your workouts, fresh and engaging workouts will keep your fitness routine stimulating.

By adhering to these principles, you will gain the knowledge needed to understand and (with a bit of experience) develop a tailored training program that aligns perfectly with your goals. This personalized approach will supercharge your results and keep your motivation soaring on your fitness journey. Remember, consistency, dedication, and the right mindset are the secret ingredients for achieving your goals!

As your "paper trainer", I am here to supporting and guiding you at every stage. Together we will create a program designed to empower you to surpass your limits and become the version of yourself. Let's dive in, wholeheartedly embrace the process, and embark on this exciting fitness adventure together!

BEGINNER'S PLANS: BUILDING A STRONG FOUNDATION

I want to congratulate you for taking the first step towards achieving a more balanced body through Wall Pilates!

In this section I am so excited to present two different three-week workout plans designed for beginners. My aim is to assist you in developing a groundwork of strength, stability and flexibility. The exercises (as well as the set-repetition progression) included in these plans have been thoughtfully chosen to focus on all key muscle groups while simultaneously improving body awareness and control.

Prepare yourself for an experience that will not only boost your physical abilities but also enhance your aesthetic wellbeing. This is just the beginning!

I suggest you to complete several times the entire two programs before jumping into the intermediate plans. In the first try keeping a rest time between each set of 60 seconds (60"); if you feel it too easy to you, decrease rests by 10 seconds at a time. If you'll be able to easily complete both workout plans with a rest time of 30" between each set, you are ready to get your toes into the intermediate plans' realm!

Discover Your Strength Workout - The Path to Radiance with Wall Pilates!

Week 1: Building Core Strength and Stability

- **Day 1:**

Wall Plank: Perform 3 sets of 30-60 seconds hold (depending on your fitness level), focusing on maintaining a strong and stable core throughout the exercise.

Wall Leg Raises: Perform 3 sets of 10-12 repetitions, targeting lower abs and hip flexor strength.

Wall Bridge: Perform 3 sets of 10-12 repetitions, engaging glutes and hamstrings for strength and activation.

- **Day 2:**

Wall Roll-Ups: Perform 3 sets of 10-12 repetitions, emphasizing abdominal control and flexibility.

Wall Bicycle Crunches: Perform 3 sets of 10-12 repetitions, engaging the entire core and alternating sides.

Wall Side Plank with Leg Lifts: Perform 3 sets of 10-12 repetitions per side, targeting oblique sculpting and hip stability.

- **Day 3:**

Wall Squats: Perform 3 sets of 10-12 repetitions, focusing on leg and glute strength.

Wall Calf Raises: Perform 3 sets of 10-12 repetitions, working on calf definition and strength.

Wall Leg Swings: Perform 3 sets of 10-12 repetitions per leg, enhancing hip mobility and stability.

Week 2: Sculpting Abs and Obliques

- **Day 1:**

Wall Push-Ups: Perform 3 sets of 10-12 repetitions, targeting chest, arm, and core strength.

Wall Triceps Push-Ups: Perform 3 sets of 10-12 repetitions, promoting arm definition and tone.

Wall Rows: Perform 3 sets of 10-12 repetitions, improving upper back strength and posture.

- **Day 2:**

Wall Lunges: Perform 3 sets of 10-12 repetitions per leg, emphasizing balance and lower body toning.

Wall Shoulder Press: Perform 3 sets of 10-12 repetitions, enhancing shoulder strength and stability.

Wall Side Crunches: Perform 3 sets of 10-12 repetitions per side, sculpting the oblique muscles.

- **Day 3:**

Wall Pike: Perform 3 sets of 10-12 repetitions, focusing on core, shoulder, and hamstring strength.

Wall Mountain Climbers: Perform 3 sets of 10-12 repetitions, improving cardiovascular endurance and core activation.

Wall Reverse Fly: Perform 3 sets of 10-12 repetitions, sculpting the upper back.

Week 3: Enhancing Lower Body Strength and Mobility

- **Day 1:**

Wall Spiderman Plank: Perform 3 sets of 10-12 repetitions, engaging the entire body and strengthening the core.

Wall Leg Swings: Perform 3 sets of 10-12 repetitions, targeting your adductors and abductors to shape your inner and outer thing.

Wall Roll-Ups: Perform 3 sets of 10-12 repetitions, focusing on abdominal control, flexibility, and strength.

- **Day 2:**

Wall Lunges: Perform 3 sets of 10-12 repetitions per leg. Focus on your lower body muscles, including the quadriceps, hamstrings, and glutes.

Wall Triceps Push-Ups: Perform 3 sets of 10-12 repetitions, promoting arm definition and tone.

Wall Bicycle Crunches: Perform 3 sets of 10-12 repetitions, engaging the entire core.

- **Day 3:**

Wall Burpees: Perform 3 sets of 10-12 repetitions, engaging the entire body for full-body conditioning and power.

Wall Pike: Perform 3 sets of 10-12 repetitions, focusing on core, shoulder, and hamstring strength.

Wall Bridge: Perform 3 sets of 10-12 repetitions, engaging glutes, hamstrings, and enhancing hip mobility.

Tips

- Focus on proper form and technique for each exercise, follow carefully the step-by-step guides we discussed in the previous chapters. Quality of movement is more important than quantity.

- To enhance the mind body connection and engage your core muscles during workouts I suggest to incorporate breathing techniques. This practice involves taking breaths that help you focus and center yourself. By inhaling and exhaling deeply you can intensify the benefits of your exercise routine.

Body Awakening Workout - Your Empowering Journey Begins on the Wall!

Week 1: Building Core Strength and Stability

- **Day 1:**

Wall Plank: Perform 3 sets of 30-60 seconds hold (depending on your fitness level), focusing on maintaining a strong and stable core throughout the exercise. This foundational exercise activates your deep abdominal muscles, providing a solid base for all movements.

Wall Leg Raises: Perform 3 sets of 10-12 repetitions, targeting lower abs and hip flexor strength. This exercise helps tone and strengthen the lower abdominal muscles and hip flexors.

Wall Bridge: Perform 3 sets of 10-12 repetitions, engaging glutes and hamstrings for strength and activation. The Wall Bridge enhances glute and hamstring activation while promoting core stability.

- **Day 2:**

Wall Roll-Ups: Perform 3 sets of 10-12 repetitions, emphasizing abdominal control and flexibility. This exercise enhances abdominal strength and improves overall flexibility.

Wall Bicycle Crunches: Perform 3 sets of 10-12 repetitions, engaging the entire core and alternating sides. This variation of traditional bicycle crunches targets both upper and lower abdominal muscles.

Wall Side Plank with Leg Lifts: Perform 3 sets of 10-12 repetitions per side, targeting oblique sculpting and hip stability. This exercise strengthens the oblique muscles and enhances lateral stability.

- **Day 3:**

Wall Squats: Perform 3 sets of 10-12 repetitions, focusing on leg and glute strength. Wall Squats target the quadriceps, hamstrings, and gluteal muscles for lower body toning.

Wall Calf Raises: Perform 3 sets of 10-12 repetitions, working on calf definition and strength. This exercise targets the calf muscles, aiding in lower leg toning.

Wall Leg Swings: Perform 3 sets of 10-12 repetitions per leg, enhancing hip mobility and stability. Wall Leg Swings help improve hip flexibility and mobility while activating the hip muscles.

Week 2: Total Body Strengthening

- **Day 1:**

Wall Push-Ups: Perform 3 sets of 10-12 repetitions, targeting chest, arm, and core strength. Wall Push-Ups engage the chest, triceps, and core muscles to enhance your upper body's tone.

Wall Triceps Push-Ups: Perform 3 sets of 10-12 repetitions, promoting arm definition and tone. This variation focuses on strengthening and sculpting the triceps.

Wall Rows: Perform 3 sets of 10-12 repetitions, improving upper back strength and posture. Wall Rows target the upper back muscles and help improve posture.

- **Day 2:**

Wall Lunges: Perform 3 sets of 10-12 repetitions per leg, emphasizing balance and lower body toning. Wall Lunges target the quadriceps, hamstrings, and glutes while enhancing balance.

Wall Shoulder Press: Perform 3 sets of 10-12 repetitions, enhancing shoulder strength and stability. This exercise focuses on the deltoid muscles for shoulder definition and arms toning.

Wall Side Crunches: Perform 3 sets of 10-12 repetitions per side, sculpting the oblique muscles. Wall Side Crunches target the obliques for a defined waistline.

- **Day 3:**

Wall Pike: Perform 3 sets of 10-12 repetitions, focusing on core, shoulder, and hamstring strength. Wall Pike strengthens the core, shoulders, and hamstrings.

Wall Mountain Climbers: Perform 3 sets of 10-12 repetitions, improving cardiovascular endurance and core activation. This dynamic exercise engages the core and boosts cardiovascular fitness.

Wall Reverse Fly: Perform 3 sets of 10-12 repetitions, sculpting the upper back. Wall Reverse Fly targets the rear deltoids and upper back muscles for improved posture.

Week 3: Enhancing Lower Body Strength and Mobility

- **Day 1:**

Wall Spiderman Plank: Perform 3 sets of 10-12 repetitions, engaging the entire body and strengthening the core. This variation of the plank exercise incorporates leg movement, challenging the core and promoting full-body engagement.

Wall Leg Swings: Perform 3 sets of 10-12 repetitions, targeting your adductors and abductors to shape your inner and outer thigh. Wall Leg Swings help enhance hip mobility and strengthen the inner and outer thigh muscles.

Wall Squats: Perform 3 sets of 10-12 repetitions, focusing on quadriceps, hamstrings, and gluteal muscles activation. Remember, this exercise will become your lower body's best friend.

- **Day 2:**

Wall Lunges: Perform 3 sets of 10-12 repetitions per leg. Focus on your lower body muscles, including the quadriceps, hamstrings, and glutes.

Wall Triceps Push-Ups: Perform 3 sets of 10-12 repetitions, promoting arm definition and tone. Continue to sculpt and strengthen the triceps.

Wall Bicycle Crunches: Perform 3 sets of 10-12 repetitions, engaging the entire core. This exercise challenges the core and obliques.

- **Day 3:**

Wall Burpees: Perform 3 sets of 10-12 repetitions, engaging the entire body for full-body conditioning and power. Wall Burpees provide a dynamic and challenging full-body workout.

Wall Pike: Perform 3 sets of 10-12 repetitions, focusing on core, shoulder, and hamstring strength. This exercise continues to target the core, shoulders, and hamstrings.

Wall Bridge: Perform 3 sets of 10-12 repetitions, engaging glutes, hamstrings, and enhancing hip mobility. Wall Bridge adds further activation to the glutes and hamstrings.

Tips

- Focus on Proper Form: During each exercise, pay close attention to your body's alignment and technique. Maintain a neutral spine, engage your core muscles, and keep your movements controlled and smooth. Proper form ensures maximum effectiveness and minimizes the risk of injury. This beginner workout routine aims to teach you the base of Wall Pilates so keep your time, don't rush and build a strong foundation!

- Listen to Your Body: While it's essential to challenge yourself, remember that everyone's fitness level is different. If an exercise feels too difficult or uncomfortable, don't hesitate to modify it or take a short break. Listen to your body's signals and progress at a pace that feels right for you. Consistency and gradual improvement will lead to incredible results over time.

Over the weeks you'll notice some amazing changes, in your body and overall well-being. This beginners Wall Pilates workout plans are designed to help you strengthen your core tone your abs and obliques and improve body strength and flexibility, giving you a solid foundation to the more advance workout plans. With effort dedication and a positive mindset, you'll be astonished by the aesthetic benefits that Pilates can bring.

Remember, this is the beginning of your Pilates journey. As you progress, don't hesitate to explore the variations I have shown you in the step-by-step guides of each exercise.

Keep pushing yourself while maintaining form and alignment. Embrace the process enjoy the journey and let Pilates transform not your body but your mind.

Prepare yourself to experience the life changing power of Wall Pilates and embrace the path towards a fitter and more vibrant version of yourself!

INTERMEDIATE WORKOUT PLANS: PROGRESSING AND CHALLENGING YOUR BODY

Congratulations on reaching the intermediate phase of your Wall Pilates journey! Here we have three different six-week workout plans tailored to intermediate level practitioners, like yourself. This plan aims to bring dynamism and progression to your routine targeting your strength, flexibility and overall body conditioning. Through a selection of exercises handpicked from the options previously discussed, you'll witness aesthetic improvements while advancing further on your fitness path. As I previously suggested for the beginner's plan, repeat several times these three workout plans before diving into the advanced program.

Let's jump in and discover the wonders these plans have in store for you!

Workout Plan Structure:

- Three workouts per week, with a rest day between each session, allowing for adequate recovery and muscle adaptation.

- Each weekly workout includes a sufficient number of exercises to stimulate all major muscle groups at least once per week, promoting balanced and comprehensive development.

- Rest 60" between each set.

Empower and Transform Workout

Week 1-2: Foundation Building

Week 1

- **Day 1:**

Wall Plank: Perform 3 sets of 60 seconds hold, focusing on maintaining a strong and stable core throughout the exercise.

Wall Squats: Complete 3 sets of 10-12 repetitions, emphasizing proper form and engaging your leg and glute muscles.

- **Day 2:**

Wall Lunges: Perform 3 sets of 10-12 repetitions per leg, focusing on controlled movement and engaging your glutes, quads and hip flexors.

Wall Shoulder Press: Complete 3 sets of 10-12 repetitions, utilizing proper form and emphasizing shoulder strength and stability.

- **Day 3:**

Wall Roll-Ups: Perform 3 sets of 8-10 repetitions, focusing on controlled movement and enhancing abdominal control and flexibility.

Wall Rows: Complete 3 sets of 10-12 repetitions, emphasizing proper form and engaging your upper back muscles.

Week 2

Follow the same workout scheme of Week 1 but:

- perform 5 sets of each exercise;

- diminish the repetitions of each exercise by 2;

- consider 30 seconds hold as a set of Wall Plank.

Example: Day 1 workout of Week 2 will be composed by 5 sets of 30 seconds hold of *Wall Plank* and 5 sets of 8-10 repetitions per set of *Wall Squats*.

Week 3-4: Increasing Intensity

Week 3

- **Day 1:**

Wall Leg Raises: Perform 4 sets of 10-12 repetitions per side, focusing on maintaining proper form and engaging your oblique and hip muscles.

Wall Lunges: Complete 3 sets of 10-12 repetitions per leg, emphasizing balance and lower body toning.

- **Day 2:**

Wall Bicycle Crunches: Perform 4 sets of 10-12 repetitions, alternating sides and focusing on total core engagement.

Wall Triceps Push-Ups: Complete 3 sets of 10-12 repetitions, utilizing proper form and targeting your triceps for definition and tone.

- **Day 3:**

Wall Bridge: Perform 4 sets of 10-12 repetitions, focusing on glute activation and hamstring strength.

Wall Reverse Fly: Complete 3 sets of 10-12 repetitions, emphasizing upper back sculpting and postural improvement.

Week 4

Follow the same workouts of Week 3 but:

- raise by 2 the sets of the first exercise of the day;

- double the sets of the second exercise;

- diminish the repetitions of each exercise by 2.

Example: Day 1 of Week 4 will be composed by 6 sets of 8-10 repetitions of *Wall Side Plank with Leg Lifts* and 6 sets of 8-10 repetitions of *Wall Lunges.*

Week 5-6: Pushing Your Limits

Week 5

- **Day 1:**

Wall Pike: Perform 4 sets of 10-12 repetitions, focusing on core, shoulder, and hamstring strength.

Wall Burpees: Complete 4 sets of 10-12 repetitions, engaging your entire body for full-body conditioning and power.

- **Day 2:**

Wall Side Crunches: Perform 4 sets of 10-12 repetitions per side, focusing on oblique sculpting and toning.

Wall Mountain Climbers: Complete 4 sets of 10-12 repetitions, emphasizing cardiovascular endurance and core activation.

- **Day 3:**

Wall Squats: Perform 4 sets of 10-12 repetitions, targeting your calf muscles for definition and strength.

Wall Spiderman Plank: Complete 4 sets of 10-12 repetitions, engaging your core and total body for strength and stability.

Week 6

Follow the same workouts of Week 5 but:

- double the sets of the first exercise of the day;

- raise by 2 the sets of the second exercise

- diminish the repetitions of each exercise by 2.

Example: Day 1 of Week 6 will be composed by 8 sets of 8-10 repetitions of *Wall Pike* and 6 sets of 8-10 repetitions of *Wall Lunges*.

Sleek and Strong Workout

Week 1-2: Strengthen and Tone

Week 1

- **Day 1:**

Wall Roll-Ups: Perform 3 sets of 8-10 repetitions, focusing on abdominal control and flexibility.

Wall Squats: Complete 4 sets of 10-12 repetitions, emphasizing proper form and engaging your leg and glute muscles.

- **Day 2:**

Wall Pike: Perform 3 sets of 10-12 repetitions, targeting core, shoulder, and hamstring strength.

Wall Side Crunches: Complete 4 sets of 10-12 repetitions per side, focusing on oblique and hip stability.

- **Day 3:**

Wall Bicycle Crunches: Perform 4 sets of 10-12 repetitions, alternating sides and engaging your total core.

Wall Triceps Push-Ups: Complete 3 sets of 10-12 repetitions, utilizing proper form and targeting your triceps for definition and tone.

Week 2

Follow the same workout scheme of Week 1 but for each exercise:

- raise the sets by 2;
- diminish the repetitions by 2.

Example: Day 1 of Week 2 will be composed by 5 sets of 8-10 reps of *Wall Roll-Ups* and 6 sets of 8-10 reps of *Wall Squats*.

Week 3-4: Power and Endurance

Week 3

- **Day 1:**

Wall Leg Swings: Perform 4 sets of 10-12 repetitions per leg, focusing on lower abs and hip flexor strength.

Wall Shoulder Press: Complete 4 sets of 10-12 repetitions, emphasizing shoulder strength and stability.

- **Day 2:**

Wall Spiderman Plank: Perform 4 sets of 10-12 repetitions, engaging your core and total body for strength and stability.

Wall Mountain Climbers: Complete 4 sets of 10-12 repetitions, emphasizing cardiovascular endurance and core activation.

- **Day 3:**

Wall Side Crunches: Perform 4 sets of 10-12 repetitions per side, focusing on oblique sculpting and toning.

Wall Rows: Complete 4 sets of 10-12 repetitions, emphasizing proper form and engaging your upper back muscles.

Week 4

Follow the same workouts of Week 3 but:

- raise by 2 the sets of the first exercise of the day;

- double the sets of the second one;

- diminish the repetitions of each exercise by 2.

Example: Day 1 of Week 4 will be composed by 6 sets of 8-10 repetitions of *Wall Leg Swings* and 8 sets of 8-10 repetitions of *Wall Shoulder Press*.

Week 5-6: Challenge and Progress

Week 5

- **Day 1:**

Wall Bridge: Perform 4 sets of 10-12 repetitions, focusing on glute activation and hamstring strength.

Wall Push-Ups: Complete 4 sets of 10-12 repetitions, engaging your chest, arms, and core.

- **Day 2:**

Wall Reverse Fly: Perform 4 sets of 10-12 repetitions, emphasizing upper back sculpting and postural improvement.

Wall Lunges: Complete 4 sets of 10-12 repetitions per leg, focusing on balance and lower body toning.

- **Day 3:**

Wall Plank: Perform 4 sets of 60 seconds hold, focusing on core activation and stability.

Wall Burpees: Complete 4 sets of 10-12 repetitions, engaging your entire body for full-body conditioning and power.

Week 6

Follow the same workouts of Week 5 but:

- double the sets of the first exercise of the day;
- raise by 2 the sets of the second exercise;
- diminish the repetitions of each exercise by 2;
- consider 45 seconds hold as one set of Wall Plank.

Example: Day 1 of Week 6 will be composed by 8 sets of 8-10 repetitions of *Wall Bridge* and 6 sets of 8-10 repetitions of *Wall Push-Ups*.

Unleash Your Inner Goddess Workout

Week 1-2: Turn on Your Body

Week 1

- **Day 1:**

Wall Side Plank: Perform 4 sets of 10-12 repetitions, focusing on obliques activation and stability.

Wall Squats: Complete 3 sets of 10-12 repetitions, engaging your leg and glute muscles for strength and toning.

- **Day 2:**

Wall Roll-Ups: Perform 4 sets of 8-10 repetitions, emphasizing abdominal control and flexibility.

Wall Reverse Fly: Complete 3 sets of 10-12 repetitions, targeting your upper back muscles for sculpting and postural improvement.

- **Day 3:**

Wall Mountain Climbers: Perform 4 sets of 10-12 repetitions, combining cardiovascular endurance with core activation.

Wall Push-Ups: Complete 3 sets of 10-12 repetitions, engaging your chest, arms, and core for strength and definition.

Week 2

Follow the same workout scheme of Week 1 but for each exercise:

- raise the sets by 1;
- raise the repetitions by 5.

Example: Day 1 of Week 2 will be composed by 5 sets of 15-17 reps of *Wall Side Plank* and 4 sets of 15-17 reps of *Wall Squats*.

Week 3-4: Adding Challenge and Complexity

Week 3

- **Day 1:**

Wall Burpees: Perform 4 sets of 10-12 repetitions per leg, focusing on lower abs and hip flexor strength.

Wall Bridge: Complete 4 sets of 10-12 repetitions, activating your glutes and hamstrings for strength and stability.

- **Day 2:**

Wall Side Crunches: Perform 4 sets of 10-12 repetitions per side, targeting your oblique muscles for sculpting and toning.

Wall Triceps Push-Ups: Complete 3 sets of 10-12 repetitions, focusing on your triceps for definition and tone.

- **Day 3:**

Wall Lunges: Perform 4 sets of 10-12 repetitions per leg, emphasizing balance and lower body toning.

Wall Rows: Complete 3 sets of 10-12 repetitions, engaging your upper back muscles for improved posture and strength.

Week 4

Follow the same workout scheme of Week 3 but:

- raise the sets by 2 in the first exercise;

- raise the repetitions by 5 in the second one.

Example: Day 1 of Week 4 will be composed by 6 sets of 10-12 reps of *Wall Burpees* and 4 sets of 15-17 reps of *Wall Bridge*.

Week 5-6: Progression and Mastery

Week 5

- **Day 1:**

Wall Lunges: Perform 3 sets of 8-10 repetitions, focusing on controlled abdominal movement and increased flexibility.

Wall Calf Raises: Complete 3 sets of 10-12 repetitions, targeting your calf muscles for definition and strength.

- **Day 2:**

Wall Push-Ups: Perform 3 sets of 10-12 repetitions, emphasizing proper form and engaging your chest, arms, and core.

Wall Spiderman Plank: Complete 3 sets of 10-12 repetitions, engaging your core and entire body for total body strength and stability.

- **Day 3:**

Wall Squats: Perform 3 sets of 10-12 repetitions per side, focusing on oblique sculpting and toning.

Wall Rows: Complete 3 sets of 10-12 repetitions, targeting your upper back muscles for improved posture and strength.

Week 6

Follow the same workout scheme of Week 5 but:

- alternate one set of the first exercise with a set of the second one (with no rest in between);

- double the sets.

Example: Day 1 of Week 4 will be composed by 6 sets of 10-12 reps of *Wall Lunges* combined with 6 sets of 10-12 reps of *Wall Calf Raises*. You have to perform your 10-12 reps per leg of *Wall Lunges*, after that without any rest, do 10-12 reps of *Wall Calf Raises* and so take your 60 seconds of rest. Repeat this 6 times.

Pay attention to maintaining form and alignment throughout each exercise taking into consideration the needs and limitations of your body.

Remember to breathe and engage your core muscles consistently during the workouts to achieve results.

To support your training and recovery make sure to nourish your body with proper meals and stay very well hydrated (*psst* check the Bonus Two at the end of the book!).

As you progress through this Wall Pilates workout plan, you'll witness transformations in your strength, flexibility and overall physique. The principle of the so called "progressive overload" ensures that you continuously challenge your body and push its limits. Embrace the journey, stay dedicated and revel in the benefits that await you.

Prepare yourself to unlock your potential redefine your boundaries and savor the results that accompany an intermediate level Wall Pilates practice. Let your inner strength radiate brightly!

Enjoy the process, celebrate your progress, and embrace the transformation that lies ahead.

You've got this!

ADVANCED WORKOUT PLAN: TAKING YOUR FITNESS TO THE NEXT LEVEL

Well done advanced level practitioners! You've entered an invigorating phase in your Wall Pilates expedition. In this segment I'm going to present my six-week advanced workout plan aimed at pushing your boundaries testing your strength and enhancing your overall fitness. Keep in mind that, depending on your fitness level, you can substitute this advanced program's exercises with the "progressions" suggested for each exercise in the previous chapters. As in any aspect of your life, Be curious!

I have meticulously curated a collection of exercises that will accompany you on a metamorphosis arming you with the means to attain optimal outcomes. The workout plan entails three sessions per week striking a sweet spot between training and recovery. Welcome to my Ignite Workout Plan!

Ignite Workout Plan™

If you have already mastered all the previous workout plans, I am delighted to introduce you to the *Ignite Workout Plan™,* a six-week program meticulously crafted to unlock your strength, power and elegance. This journey is tailored to those, with a fitness level aiming to awaken every aspect of your being – body, mind and soul – propelling you towards physical prowess.

Prepare yourself for a journey of sculpting and refining your muscles enhancing your endurance and embracing the true life changing potential of Wall Pilates.

Throughout this program you will engage in three invigorating workouts each week that are guaranteed to test your limits while simultaneously inspiring and revitalising you. As you complete each session a tremendous sense of accomplishment and renewed vitality will accompany you.

It's time to let your true self blossom!

Workout Plan Structure:

- Three workouts per week, with a rest day between each session, allowing for adequate recovery and muscle adaptation.

- Each weekly workout includes a sufficient number of exercises to stimulate all major muscle groups at least once per week, promoting balanced and comprehensive development.

- Rest 60" between each set.

- High-intensity and high-volume program, to ensure you are properly conditioned, you should have been able to complete the intermediate programs before trying it.

Week 1-2: Building Strength and Endurance

Week 1

- **Day 1:**

Wall Squats: 6 sets of 10-12 repetitions for leg and glute strength.

Wall Push-Ups: 4 sets of 10-12 repetitions for chest, arm, and core strength.

Wall Spiderman Plank: 5 sets of 10-12 repetitions for total body engagement and core strength.

- **Day 2:**

Wall Bridge: 6 sets of 10-12 repetitions for glute activation and hamstring strength.

Wall Rows: 5 sets of 10-12 repetitions for upper back and posture improvement.

Wall Shoulder Press: 4 sets of 10-12 repetitions for shoulder strength and stability.

- **Day 3:**

Wall Pike: 4 sets of 10-12 repetitions for core, shoulder, and hamstring strength.

Wall Mountain Climbers: 6 sets of 10-12 repetitions for cardiovascular endurance and core activation.

Wall Side Plank with Leg Lifts: 5 sets of 10-12 repetitions for oblique and hip stability.

Week 2

Follow the same workout scheme of Week 1 but:

- For each 6-sets exercise of Week 1, raise by 2 the sets and diminish the repetitions by 2;
- For each 5-sets exercise of Week 1, raise by 1 the sets and diminish the repetitions by 2;
- For each 4-sets exercise of Week 1, raise the repetitions by 5;

Example: Day 1 of Week 2 will be composed by 8 sets of 8-10 reps of *Wall Squats*, 4 sets of 13-15 reps of *Wall Push-Ups* and 6 sets of 8-10 reps of *Wall Spiderman Plank*.

Week 3-4: Adding Complexity and Challenge

Week 3

- **Day 1:**

Wall Lunges: 3 sets of 15-20 repetitions for balance and lower body toning.

Wall Triceps Push-Ups: 4 sets of 8-10 repetitions for arm definition and tone.

Wall Reverse Fly: 4 sets of 8-10 repetitions for upper back sculpting.

- **Day 2:**

Wall Roll-Ups: 3 sets of 15-20 repetitions for abdominal control and flexibility.

Wall Bicycle Crunches: 4 sets of 8-10 repetitions for total core engagement.

Wall Leg Swings: 4 sets of 8-10 repetitions for hip mobility and stability.

- **Day 3:**

Wall Burpees: 3 sets of 15-20 repetitions for full-body conditioning.

Wall Side Crunches: 4 sets of 8-10 repetitions for oblique sculpting.

Wall Calf Raises: 3 sets of 15-20 repetitions for calf definition and strength.

Week 4

Follow the same workout scheme of Week 3 but:

- for each 3-sets exercise of Week 3, raise by 2 the sets keeping the same repetition range;

- for each 4-sets exercise of Week 3, diminish by 1 the total sets and perform 15-20 repetitions;

- diminish the rest time between sets by 15 seconds.

Example: Day 1 of Week 4 will be composed by 6 sets of 15-20 reps of *Wall Lunges,* 3 sets of 15-20 reps of *Wall Triceps Push-Ups* and 3 sets of 15-20 reps of *Wall Reverse Fly.* The rest between sets of each exercise is 45 seconds.

Week 5-6: Progression and Mastery

Week 5

- **Day 1:**

Wall Squats: 6 sets of 20 repetitions for increased leg and glute strength.

Wall Push-Ups: 4 sets of 10-12 repetitions for advanced chest, arm, and core strength.

Wall Rows: 4 sets of 10-12 repetitions for advanced core, shoulder, and hamstring strength.

- **Day 2:**

Wall Bridge: 6 sets of 20 repetitions for advanced glute activation and hamstring strength.

Wall Mountain Climbers: 4 sets of 10-12 repetitions for advanced cardiovascular endurance and core activation.

Wall Side Plank: 4 sets of 10-12 repetitions for advanced oblique and hip stability.

- **Day 3:**

Wall Burpees: 6 sets of 20 repetitions for advanced abdominal control and flexibility.

Wall Bicycle Crunches: 4 sets of 10-12 repetitions for advanced total core engagement.

Wall Leg Swings: 4 sets of 10-12 repetitions for advanced hip mobility and stability.

Week 6 (it's time to level-up my girl!)

Follow the same workout scheme of Week 5 but:

- For each 6-sets exercise of Week 5, double the sets, halve the reps and diminish the rest time between sets keeping it equal to 10 seconds;

- For each 4-sets exercise of Week 5, raise by 1 the total sets, diminish the rest time between sets keeping it equal to 30 seconds keeping the same repetition range.

Example: Day 1 of Week 6 will be composed by 12 sets of 10 reps of *Wall Squats* with a 10" rest between sets; 5 sets of 10-12 reps of *Wall Push-Ups* with a 30" rest between sets and 5 sets of 10-12 reps of *Wall Rows* with a 30" rest between sets.

As an advanced-level practitioner, continue to challenge yourself by increasing resistance, range of motion, or intensity of exercises over time.

Feel free to repeat the *Ignite Workout Plan™* many times, it's not a mandatory 6-weeks program. If you want to experiment different progression, you can try repeating it raising the repetitions, the sets or diminishing the rest time between the sets. Experiment the progression type you enjoy the most!

One above all, maintain proper form and alignment throughout each movement, focusing on quality over quantity. As I stated in the Workout Plan Structure, this program is designed to be very intense and demanding. If you plan on repeating it times in a row, I recommend incorporating an Intermediate Plan for one week in between each repetition.

To ensure understanding, once you have finished the 6 week *Ignite Workout Plan™* (or at the latest after completing it twice in a row); select the first week workout plan from your preferred Intermediate Plan and complete it before attempting another round of the *Ignite Workout Plan™*. This will allow your body to recover effectively.

Listen to your body and adjust the workout plan as needed to prevent overexertion and ensure proper recovery.

Incorporate active rest days and include stretching exercises to maintain flexibility and prevent muscle imbalances.

BONUS ONE! GLUTE GODDESS™

SCULPT AND TONE PERFECT ABS AND BOOTY

Thank you for joining me in this bonus chapter! Here we will delve into a Wall Pilates workout regimen tailor made to sculpt a stunning abs and booty. This program focuses on these regions to assist you in developing a flat and aesthetic belly and achieving well-toned juicy booty!

Notice that this is an advanced level program, I kindly suggest you to properly condition yourself with the intermediate programs before trying to attempt *Glute Goddess™* Program.

Prepare yourself for a six-week adventure that will push your limits and bring about changes, in your physique leaving you with a sense of confidence and empowerment.

Are you prepared to embrace the effects of wall Pilates resulting in abs and a captivating derrière? Let's get started!

Week 1-2: Ignite the Spark

Week 1

- **Day 1:**

Wall Plank: Perform 3 sets of 75 seconds hold, focusing on core activation and stability. Rest 45" between sets.

Wall Squats: Complete 3 sets of 10-12 repetitions, emphasizing leg and glute strength. Rest 45" between sets.

- **Day 2:**

Wall Lunges: Perform 3 sets of 10-12 repetitions per leg, targeting your quads, hamstrings and glutes. Rest 45" between sets.

Wall Bridge: Complete 3 sets of 10-12 repetitions, activating your glutes and hamstrings. Rest 45" between sets.

- **Day 3:**

Wall Bicycle Crunches: Perform 3 sets of 10-12 repetitions, engaging your total core. Rest 45" between sets.

Wall Lunges: Complete 3 sets of 10-12 repetitions per leg, focusing on balance and lower body toning. Rest 45" between sets.

Week 2

Follow the same workout scheme as Week 1 but:

- perform 5 sets of each exercise;

- decrease the repetitions of each exercise by 2;

- the scheduled sets of Wall Plank are 60 seconds instead of 75 seconds;

- add at the end of each workout one set to failure of Wall Plank.

Example: Day 1 of Week 2 will be composed by 5 sets of 60 seconds hold of *Wall Plank;* 5 sets of 8-10 reps of *Wall Squats* and one set of *Wall Plank* to failure (hold the position as long as possible, until you can't take it anymore).

Week 3-4: Power and Sculpt

Week 3

- **Day 1:**

Wall Side Plank with Leg Lifts: Perform 4 sets of 10-12 repetitions per side, focusing on oblique and hip stability. Rest 45" between sets.

Wall Spiderman Plank: Complete 4 sets of 10-12 repetitions, engaging your core and total body. Rest 45" between sets.

- **Day 2:**

Wall Side Crunches: Perform 4 sets of 10-12 repetitions per side, targeting oblique sculpting and toning. Rest 45" between sets.

Wall Shoulder Press: Complete 4 sets of 10-12 repetitions, emphasizing shoulder strength and stability. Rest 45" between sets.

- **Day 3:**

Wall Pike: Perform 4 sets of 10-12 repetitions, targeting core, shoulder, and hamstring strength. Rest 45" between sets.

Wall Mountain Climbers: Complete 4 sets of 10-12 repetitions, emphasizing cardiovascular endurance and core activation. Rest 45" between sets.

Week 4

Follow the same workouts as Week 3 but increase the intensity:

- increase the sets of the first exercise of each day by 2;

- double the sets of the second exercise;

- decrease the repetitions of each exercise by 2;

- add at the end of each workout two set to failure of Wall Burpees with 75 seconds rest between these two sets.

Example: Day 1 of Week 4 will be composed by 6 sets of 8-10 reps of *Wall Side Plank with Leg Lifts*; 8 sets of 8-10 reps of *Wall Squats* and two set of *Wall Burpees* to failure (do as many reps as possible, until you can't take it anymore).

Week 5-6: Challenge and Transform

Week 5

- **Day 1:**

Wall Burpees: Complete 4 sets of 12-15 repetitions, engaging your entire body for full-body conditioning and power. Rest 45" between sets.

Wall Leg Raises: Perform 4 sets of 10-12 repetitions, focusing on abdominal control and flexibility. Rest 45" between sets.

- **Day 2:**

Wall Squats: Complete 4 sets of 12-15 repetitions, targeting core, shoulder, and hamstring strength. Rest 45" between sets.

Wall Bicycle Crunches: Perform 4 sets of 12-15 repetitions, emphasizing proper form and feeling the burning sensation in your core. Rest 45" between sets.

- **Day 3:**

Wall Bridge: Complete 4 sets of 12-15 repetitions, sculpting your upper back and improving posture. Rest 45" between sets.

Wall Calf Raises: Perform 4 sets of 12-15 repetitions, focusing on calf definition and strength. Rest 45" between sets.

Week 6 (it will BURN)

Follow the same workouts as Week 5 but let's skyrocket the intensity!

- double the sets of the first exercise of each day;

- increase the sets of the second one by 2;

- add at the end of each workout one set to failure of Wall Squats;

- add at the end of each workout one set to failure of Wall Bridge.

Example: Day 1 of Week 6 will be composed by 8 sets of 12-15 reps of Wall Burpees; 6 sets of 12-15 reps of Wall Leg Raises; one set to failure of Wall Squats and one set to failure of Wall Bridge.

Congratulations, on completing the *Glute Goddess™* workout plan! You've embarked on a journey to strengthen and shape your muscles and glutes unlocking your inner power.

As always, I remember how much it's important to maintain consistency and dedication in order to reach your fitness goals.

Remember, the path to achieving toned abs and a fabulous booty is a process and by following this workout plan you've taken a significant step towards your ultimate fitness aspirations. Stay motivated stay committed and continue striving for greatness.

Get ready to embrace results and relish the confidence in your body!

CONCLUSION: YOUR TRANSFORMATION CONTINUES

Congratulations, my dear, on completing your journey through "Wall Pilates Workouts for Women". Just think how far you have come and how much you have discovered about yourself along the way. Throughout this book we have explored the world of Wall Pilates together uncovering its advantages trying out exercises that target various muscle groups and challenging progressive workout plans tailored to your fitness level. Now as we reach the end of this adventure with Wall Pilates it's important to remember that your transformation is a commitment to your health and overall wellness.

Wall Pilates has proven itself to be an exercise method that engages both your body and mind. By incorporating it into your fitness routine you have not strengthened your core, sculpted your muscles and enhanced your flexibility; but also developed discipline, resilience and self-confidence. You have experienced first-hand the changes that occur when you prioritize your well-being and invest in yourself!

However, this is not the end, it signifies the beginning of a chapter in your fitness journey. The knowledge and skills you have gained from this book will serve as a foundation for a lifetime of mental well-being. Take pride in the progress you have achieved the inches you have shed and the newfound vitality that emanates from within. Let these accomplishments ignite your motivation and spur you to keep striving for greatness.

Remember fitness is a pursuit that encompasses more than exercise. It involves nurturing your body through nutrition, ample rest and self-care. Embrace a rounded lifestyle that nourishes your body and nurtures your soul. Surround yourself with influences seek guidance from experts and find pleasure in the journey; celebrate each triumph, learn from setbacks as they are essential experiences that foster growth and development.

While reflecting on your transformation hold onto the words of the American poet Maya Angelou: *"Nothing can dim the radiance that emanates from, within"*. You have discovered your strength, which permeates every movement, every breath and every decision you make. Carry this light as you continue on your fitness voyage inspiring others through your commitment, resilience and unwavering self-belief.

With love and boundless enthusiasm,

[*Aurora Powers*]

BONUS TWO! 28-DAYS DIET PLAN

Hey, we are not done yet! Our journey is far from over, it's time to kick things up a notch and ensure those hard-won results become your lifelong story of strength and confidence. Get ready to discover a treasure trove of strategies that will not only help you maintain your progress but will also light up your life with vitality and well-being that radiate from within. Ready to dive in?

As you've embraced the power of movement, it's equally essential to fuel your body with the right nutrients. Picture this: a plate adorned with an array of vibrant, colorful fruits and veggies, accompanied by lean proteins, whole grains, and the right fats to keep your energy soaring. And let's not forget the hydration, a constant stream of water that keeps your body's engines revving. Now, let's agree to bid adieu to those processed snacks and sugary temptations – your body deserves the best, and you're here to deliver!

But here's the golden nugget: a 28-day diet plan that's your passport to a world of delectable and health-boosting cuisine. How do you get your hands on it? Simple, just give that QR code below a scan, and voilà, you're on your way to fit-culinary nirvana!

Imagine having a curated guide that takes the guesswork out of your daily meals. This isn't just a diet plan; it's your first personal roadmap to a journey where food becomes your ally, and nourishing your body is a joyful act of self-love.

So, are you ready to embark on this flavorful adventure? See this QR code as your gateway to a world where nutrition and fitness unite in a harmonious dance, creating a symphony of wellness that sings your praises!

As I extend my heartfelt thanks for joining me on this journey, know that you, my readers, are the heartbeat of this endeavor. Without you, this book is just words on paper; with you, it becomes a dynamic wellspring of inspiration, igniting my motivation. Consider this my heartfelt expression of gratitude.

See you on the other side, where radiant vitality is your new norm,

[*Aurora Powers*]

Made in the USA
Columbia, SC
24 May 2024

36160103R00052